GETTING STRONG

Developing Your Chest

GETTING STRONG

Developing Your Chest

by Mark Reifkind

ANDERSON WORLD
BOOKS, INC.

Library of Congress Cataloging in Publication Data

Reifkind, Mark, 1957-
Developing your chest.

(The Getting Strong book series ; bk. 3)
1. Chest. 2. Exercise. 3. Weight lifting. I. Title.
II. Series.
GV508.R45 1984 796.4'1 84-16904
ISBN 0-89037-306-X

Cover photo by Geoffrey Baris
Exercise sequence photos are by Kevin Auyong; other photos are by Greg Aiken, Alex Antuck, Garry Bartlett, William Heimanson, David Keith and Robert Spector.

Exercise sequence photos were taken at Iron Dynamics in Mountain View, California.

Anderson World Books, Inc.
1400 Stierlin Road, Mountain View, CA 94043

CONTENTS

To Arnold Schwarzenegger, whose physique inspired me to begin bodybuilding, and whose image still keeps me inspired through many long, hard and sometimes discouraging training sessions.

ONE: CHEST CHAMPIONS

The chest muscles are probably the second most highly trained muscles, next to the biceps, of course. These large muscles clearly show on a person who has trained with weights. Think of the people you know with shallow, sunken chests. Do you think of them as strong and powerful? It's not likely.

The chest is the muscle of the bear and symbolizes power and strength to most people, especially athletes. They know that someone with a strong chest usually has a strong and powerful upper body as well. The exercises you use to train the chest can involve a lot of weight and be a challenge. The Bench Press is probably the most popular exercise in the gym. Go into any gym at any time of the day and you will see people benching. Even more so than curls, the Bench Press holds a special place in the hearts of athletes.

As the centerpiece of the physique, the chest sets off the rest of the body. If the center of your physique is flat, sunken and unimpressive, it's not going to help make a strong initial impression. A chest and rib cage (an important part of the chest area) that lifts up and out, and is tight and strong, will attract attention.

Training the chest is quite satisfying because as one of the larger body parts (the big three are chest, back and legs) it pumps up well. Other than the arms, the chest is probably the most satisfying pump you can get.

I teach bodybuilding for a living, and almost everyone I train, men and women, tell me that the chest is the main area they want to build. There are other body parts and areas they want to work on, but the chest is always included.

Developing the chest is no simple task. The chest is made of up many muscles that must be trained for size, shape, symmetry and balance to look right.

A lot of people who come to me for advice want to train just one area of their body. They'll tell me, "I just want to build my arms or my legs." I tell them this is fine, but I remind them it's important to always train all the muscles of the body, even if they want to improve only one area. Training only one part of the body can lead to muscle imbalances, which invites injury.

By building a solid foundation, there's less chance of setting yourself up for injury while you're specializing on a certain muscle group. I don't advise specialization work until a person has plenty of muscle over the entire body. Working on the entire body will give you an idea what muscle groups grow fastest and what muscles grow more slowly.

In order to train the chest to its maximum, you have to isolate the pectorals from the rest of the torso muscles; you have to feel the muscle contracting. That's why it's important to use moderate poundage that allows you to concentrate on the muscle contracting. You don't want to use weights so heavy that you're barely surviving the lift.

The more you know about the anatomy of the chest, the easier it will be to visualize the muscles working. Seeing the muscle you are working in your mind's eye enhances the lift. It's true! You are tuning into your neuromuscular pathway, which the brain uses to tell the muscles what to do. As your awareness of this pathway increases, your ability to contract will improve with it.

The main chest muscle group, the pectoralis major, is usually referred to as the chest. This is really the lower part of the chest, and is called the sternal portion. The upper pectoral muscles (pecs) are called the pectoralis minor and attach to the clavicle (collarbone). The rib cage is included here because of its role in displaying the pecs. Pecs alone do not a chest make. An expanded rib cage can provide the underlying structure to set the pecs off. Just look at any of the best bodybuilders—like Arnold Schwarzenegger, Samir Bannout or Carla Dunlap—they all have magnificently developed rib cages and great pecs.

The rib cage consists of 12 ribs, 10 of which attach in the front to the sternum and in the rear to the spine. Two are called floating ribs and are attached only to the spine. The area where the rib cage attaches to the sternum consists of cartilage. This area can lengthen and expand if you do deep-breathing and stretching exercises while your body is growing. Heavy high-rep squats super-setted with dumbbell or barbell straight arm pullovers can also help to open the rib cage.

There is some controversy, however, whether adults can expand their rib cage. Some bodybuilders who believe it's possible have reported increases of up to two inches, even when they're in their forties! Science will say this is bunk. Doctors tell us that after we stop growing, the cartilage hardens and cannot stretch. Training with high reps to expand the rib cage and doing pullovers to stretch them may or may not work for adults, but even if it doesn't, you'll still gain muscle and size in the rib cage that can easily be mistaken for "chest depth."

Young or old, everyone can benefit from rib cage programs. If you are a beginning bodybuilder, you must build a core strength foundation with high-rep squats and pullovers, especially if competition is a goal.

Below the rib cage and chest cavity is the diaphragm, an umbrella-shaped muscle that separates the abdominals (we'll call them abs) and the chest cavity. It expands and contracts when you breathe, so rib cage expansion and chest training give it a good workout. The upper abs and serratus tie in nicely with the pecs and rib cage to a create an almost regal look. Carla Dunlap's rib cage and chest is a perfect example. Fully developed pecs with a strong rib cage set off the entire physique.

MUSCLE USE IN ATHLETICS AND OTHER ACTIVITIES

The chest doesn't get a specific workout from most sports activities. Nature designed the muscles to work in concert. The chest muscles are pushing muscles and work in tandem with the shoulders (deltoids) and triceps.

Gymnastics

Gymnastics probably isolates the chest muscles more than any other sport. The chest development of ring specialists is remarkable. A lot of bodybuilders, like Charles Glass (University of California, Berkeley, graduate), a Mr. America and Mr. Universe (middleweight) winner, participated in gymnastics prior to their bodybuilding careers. Jim Sietzer, Mr. Ohio and a competitor at the Mr. America many times, was also a successful all-around gymnast at the University of Ohio.

Gymnastics training relies heavily on the pecs. The parallel bars and the rings require extensive chest power. Swinging on the pommel horse and horizontal bars uses the pecs to help stabilize the torso.

Mike Silverman, a gymnast at Temple University in the 1970s, had magnificent upper torso development, especially in his chest and shoulders. They were huge, striated and ripped. The constant tension on the muscles from thousands and thousands of dips and presses on the rings had given Silverman muscularity and detail usually found at the highest levels of competitive bodybuilding.

Gymnastic training can improve your chest development, or chest training can help your gymnastics. Either way, you're bound to have a better chest.

Martial Arts

If you think martial artists don't have to use their chests much, look at any picture of Bruce Lee's. Muscle tension, punching and blocking bring the pecs of many experts of the martial arts up to the level of bodybuilders. Although some martial arts experts lift weights, many do not and yet they maintain excellent pecs. Katas (form exercises) are done with precise, controlled movements, breath control, and isometric muscle tension to stress the pecs. Kata will not increase chest size markedly, but training this way will enhance definition and muscle separation, as well as upper torso movement.

Wrestling

I have never seen a wrestler that did not have good pec development. I had the opportunity to train at the University of Iowa as a gymnast while the university's wrestling team was winning one national championship after another. The entire team had great pecs. The constant pulling, pushing and tension in wrestling develops the chest and torso muscles in a manner that weights alone could never do.

The nature of the sport plays a key role in keeping the wrestler's pecs hard and muscular. Almost all muscle groups will respond well to isometric tension and dynamic movements common to wrestling. When the pecs are overly large and without muscularity, they look fat.

Triathloning

Triathlon training (swimming, cycling, running) involves considerable use of the chest muscles in swimming. Swimmers are noted for their chest development, especially those who specialize in the breast and butterfly strokes. All those hours in the pool pay off with separation and growth of the pectorals. Triathletes also must use their

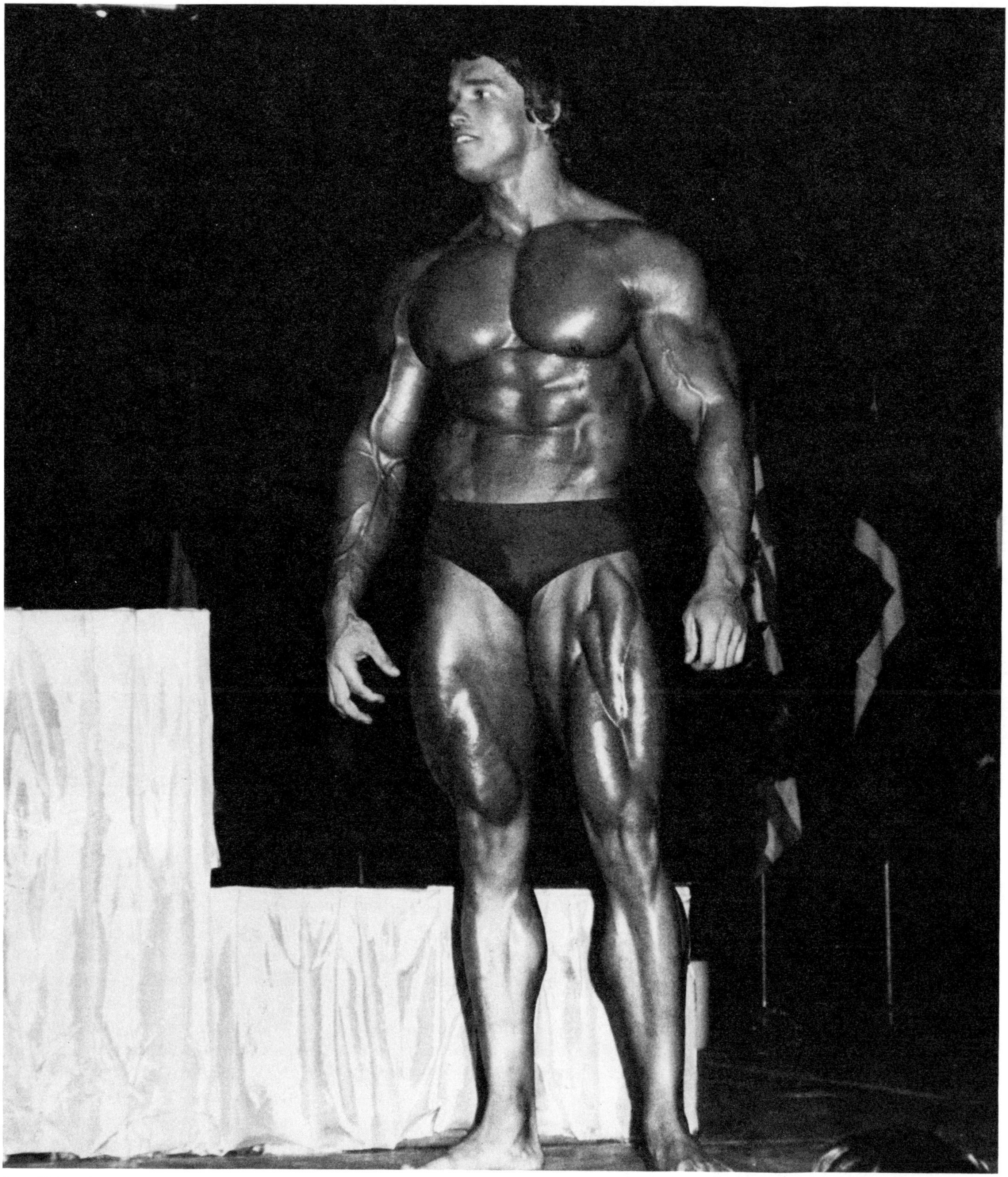

It will be a long time before another bodybuilder comes along to rival the great Arnold Schwarzenegger, seven-time Mr. Olympia. Schwarzenegger's massive chest has always been one of his strong points, but his success as a bodybuilder was in his ideal combination of size, shape and muscle symmetry. Schwarzenegger awaits the announcement of his 1974 Mr. Olympia victory.

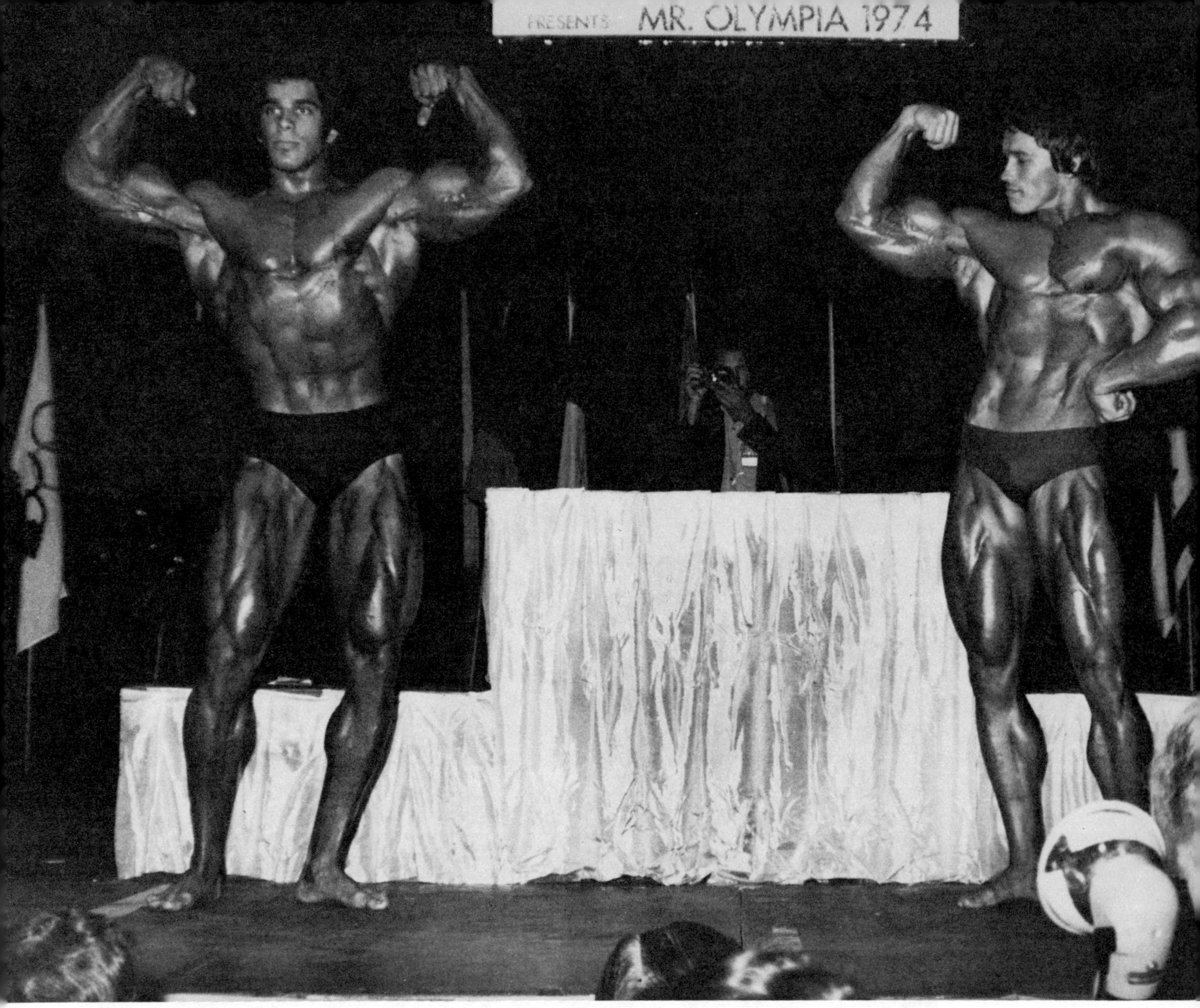

The 1970s saw some of the greatest bodybuilding competition ever, including battles between two of the best—and most famous—bodybuilders in the world, Lou Ferrigno and Arnold Schwarzenegger.

chest muscles while climbing hills on the bike, and to a lesser extent while running for upper body stabilization.

Football

The chest muscles work best in tandem with the other pushing muscles, the deltoids and triceps. This type of pushing action is extremely important in football for the linemen. Offensive linemen continually use their chests to block charging tackles and linebackers. Linebackers, who specialize in swatting their opponents into the ground, utilize the chest's main function of drawing the arms across the body. The chest muscles are also important for quarterbacks when they throw the ball. Weight work for the chest is an important part of any serious football player's training program.

Powerlifting and Bodybuilding

Needless to say, there is no other activity that will build, shape, define and strengthen the muscles of the chest and upper torso like bodybuilding and powerlifting. Powerlifting's most visible activity is the Bench Press. Powerlifters need the shoulder stability that intense chest training gives, as well as the pectoral power to blast big weights. A strong chest/torso area is also essential for stabilizing the upper body while squatting and deadlifting.

Powerlifters train to isolate the pecs with bodybuilding movements and high repetition work. They use dumbbells because they give the pecs a better stretch. Shoulder and arm work is done to increase the strength of these assisting muscles. Here is a key point for gaining size in the chest: Use a variety of exercises, techniques and training styles, to strengthen the individual pecs as well as all the surrounding, stabilizing muscles of the torso.

Bodybuilders, as we will discuss in detail, spend many hours of their training time working the chest—from every conceivable angle and with every technique available. Shape, size, symmetry, muscularity and definition all require different stress to bring out the desired adaptations. The bodybuilder's job is difficult and detailed, but the results give the greatest rewards possible. The knowledge that you have to control how you look, build, shape and mold your pecs, more than makes up for the discipline and hard work bodybuilding requires.

THE IDEAL PECS

Beauty, it is said, is in the eye of the beholder. Each person has his own idea of perfection. To some, a very large and muscular chest epitomizes strength, virility and power. That would be the perfect chest for someone. Others believe definition, muscularity and proportion to be more important than sheer size. Neither opinion is wrong.

Each person is endowed with a certain amount of potential muscle fibers, lengths of tendons and muscle bellies, neurological ability and strength. This means that nobody is going to build the exact same chest as anyone else. Each chest will be its own masterpiece, or, as bodybuilder Rory Leidermeyer says, "its own version of body perfection."

We can categorize, though, the more famous and envied chest types of such athletes as Arnold Schwarzenegger, Steve Reeves, Frank Zane and Franco Columbu.

Let's begin with the gold standard in chest development—Arnold Schwarzenegger. Virtually any photo of Schwarzenegger in his prime (early 1970s) will show you what many experts consider the epitome of male chest development: a structure that was huge but beautifully shaped, pecs that were inhumanly large but looked as if carved from stone. He had a perfect balance between the upper and lower pecs and inner pec development that was awesome.

Other bodybuilders that have basically the same pec development as Schwarzenegger are Samir Bannout, Lou Ferrigno and Tom Platz.

These men are very large, but their proportions are such that they appear fluid and well-shaped, never bulky or awkward. They all did basic exercises with barbells, dumbbells and cables to achieve their physiques. Almost everyone did dips for the chest. They did flyes to stretch the pecs and cable work for peak contractions.

Former Mr. Olympia Frank Zane has never strived for the massive muscle size that seems so natural on such bodybuilders as Lou Ferrigno and Franco Columbu. Instead, Zane has worked on perfecting his symmetry and keeping his development proportional.

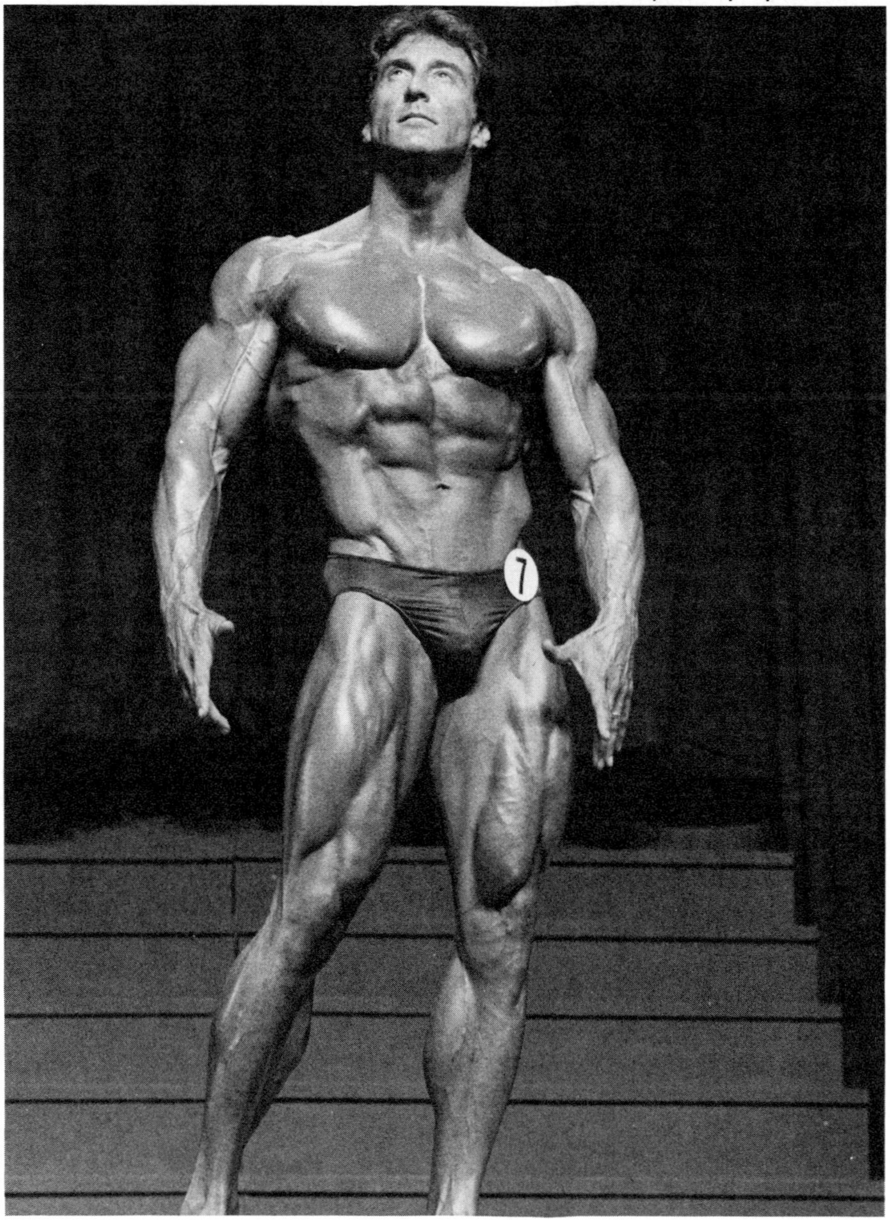

His massive symmetry is what made Schwarzenegger so acceptable to the public. He was huge but so symmetrical he didn't look awkward. Schwarzenegger says that his size was a direct result of his training methods—high reps and leverage movements like flyes that stretch and open the pectorals after they've been contracted with the various forms of barbell bench pressing.

Frank Zane, though, comes from another school of pectoral training and is a prime example of those bodybuilders who train for proportion, muscularity and symmetry rather than for huge mass and size. Schwarzenegger wanted it all—size and shape. Zane prefers his chest "lean, wide, flaring and striated," because he believes overly large pectorals detract from the arms and shoulders and give the athlete a "feminine" look. The athletic appearance is important, Zane says, and large pecs are rarely found on athletes. Muscular and well-defined pectorals are common among gymnasts and wrestlers, but massive size is rare.

Zane says he likes square pecs with density, muscularity and definition so clear that the skin appears transparent. His upper pectoral muscles are slightly smaller than the lower ones, but have excellent separation and definition. Thousands of striations appear along the inner clavicle and sternal regions, the sign of ultimate muscularity. Zane's rib cage is fairly large and muscular, and, like the rest of him, extremely well-shaped and proportionate. Zane purposely gives up some size to focus more on creating the perfect shape.

Franco Columbu's chest, on the other hand, seems like a cross between Zane's and Schwarzenegger's. Massively muscular, but with flowing lines evident even at rest, Franco's chest was state-of-the-art.

Capable of 500-pound Bench Presses, Columbu reportedly trained as fast and heavy as possible. Combining power training methods with strict bodybuilding technique, Columbu built a chest of granite.

Serge Nubret of France was an example of the European style of chest development. Focusing almost entirely on form and shape, Nubret uses very light weight for high sets and reps. Nubret uses concentration on the contraction almost entirely to the exclusion of heavy weights, which, he believes, lets him concentrate on shaping the chest muscles to their maximum. He says he can direct the contractions directly to the area that needs work. His size comes from a strength training background. The muscularity comes from the tension Nubret builds into each rep of each set. He flexes with the weights while focusing only on the muscles in contraction.

Another name associated with ideal pecs is Robby Robinson. Robinson's pec/delt tie-in and upper pec development are unearthly. The muscularity and density, along with beautifully flowing lines and complete tie-ins to all the torso muscles have made his chest a legend among bodybuilders.

A chapter on the perfect pecs would not be complete without mention of Steve Reeves. Long believed to have the perfect male body, Reeves had the square, hard pecs that Zane admires so much. He was also genetically blessed with a perfectly straight line across the bottom of his pectoral muscles, separating them from the abdominals with a slash of muscle. He used moderate weights and strict form but took each set to the end. Naturally strong, Reeves was said to deadlift 400 pounds by the ends of reverse plates!

Reeves did not have the density of a Schwarzenegger, but he was thick and massive. His incredible proportions and symmetry caused him to look much bigger than he was, the illusion of the perfectly symmetrical body.

To try to categorize all chest types here would be futile. There are as many different chest types as there are bodybuilders. Many of the top pros, past and present, had awesome chests. Train your pecs for their best combination of size, shape, symmetry, muscularity and density and you can't go wrong. Develop your own version of the perfect chest.

THE PERFECT WOMAN'S CHEST

Women bodybuilders are coming into their own in the world of physique competition. They've proven they have enough intensity and dedication to training to embarrass a lot of men trainers! Many women have discovered that training the chest and back is the easiest and also the best way to enhance the size of the bust. Building the upper pecs helps lift the breasts.

Many women who take up or desire to take up bodybuilding are afraid of losing their breast size. They have seen the competitive women bodybuilders in magazines and on television who have lost breast tissue from extensive dieting.

Intense dieting for prolonged periods causes your body to burn fat for fuel, and the breast is composed almost entirely of adipose (fat) tissue. Returning to a normal diet doesn't always bring the fat back in the same places either. If you lose breast tissue from severe dieting, it might not return when you begin eating normally again.

But I'm supposed to be convincing you of the benefits of chest training. That's why I'm telling you that training the chest with regular bodybuilding techniques and exercises doesn't cause breast tissue reduction; rather, dieting down to very low body fat levels causes this phenomenon.

If you are a competitor, you will have to lose body fat very slowly. Increase your calorie loss by adding more aerobic exercise. Train it off.

If you are not or don't plan to be a competitor, don't worry about your weight. Keep your calories high enough to train without putting on body fat and you will gain muscle without losing breast tissue. Create the perfect shape through intelligent, hard work and your chest will respond.

Women's muscular chest development is as varied as men's. Carla Dunlap and Tina Plankinger typify the muscular side. Both women have thick, striated, separated and balanced pectoral muscles. The inner pecs are extremely well-defined and muscular and give their physiques force and power.

Heavy chest training is a vital component of upper body development for women. Women carry much of their weight, size and strength in their hips and thighs. Pound for pound, an untrained woman's legs are approximately as strong as an untrained male's. Upper body strength comparisons are a different story; men are naturally stronger than women here.

For you to gain size, your upper body has to be trained diligently. Absolutely vital are pressing movements for the chest and shoulders. Flat, incline and decline bench presses with bar or dumbbell

Janice Regain is one of many women proving that muscles can be beautiful and feminine. Her well-developed chest balances the thick muscularity of her arms and shoulders.

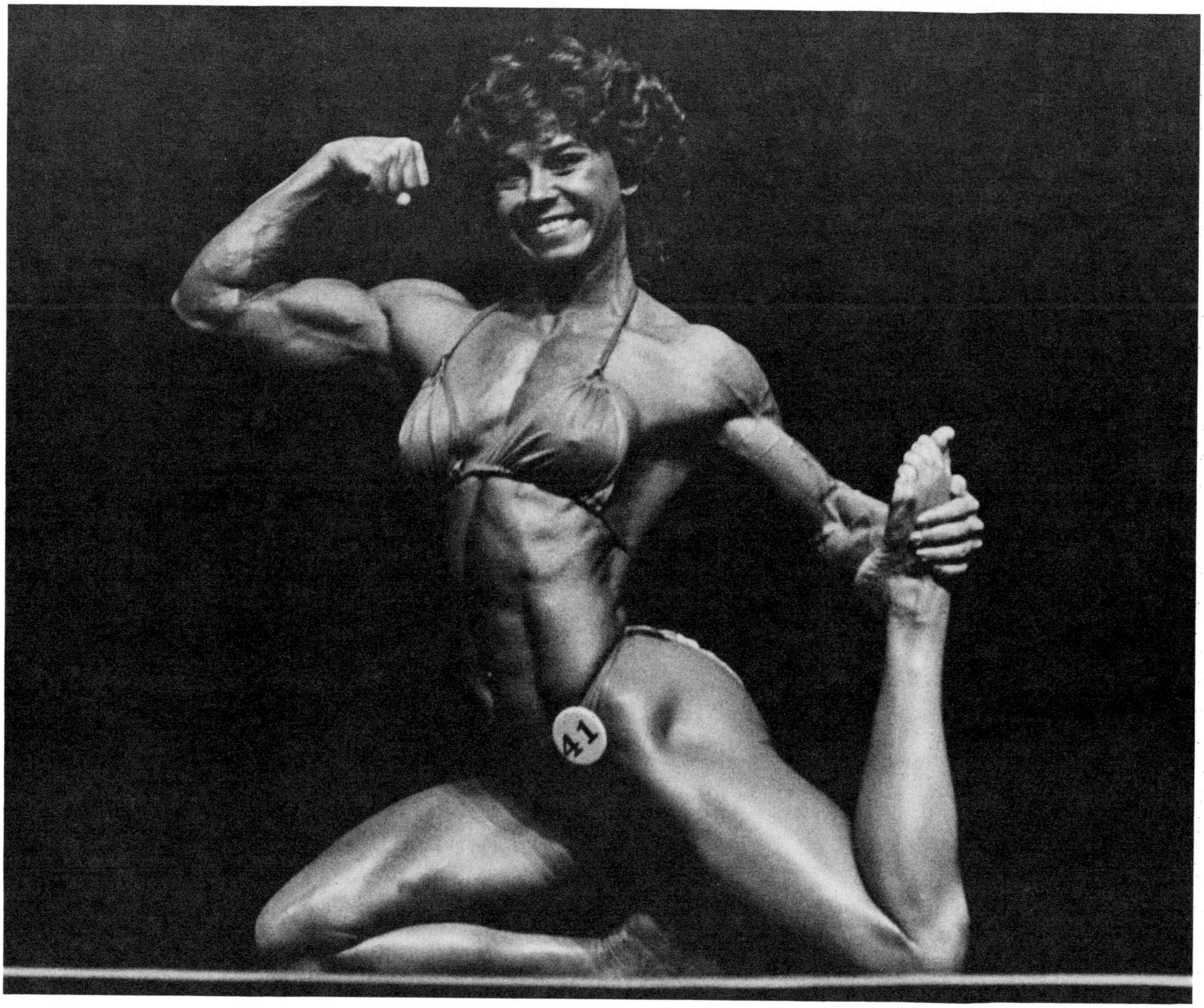

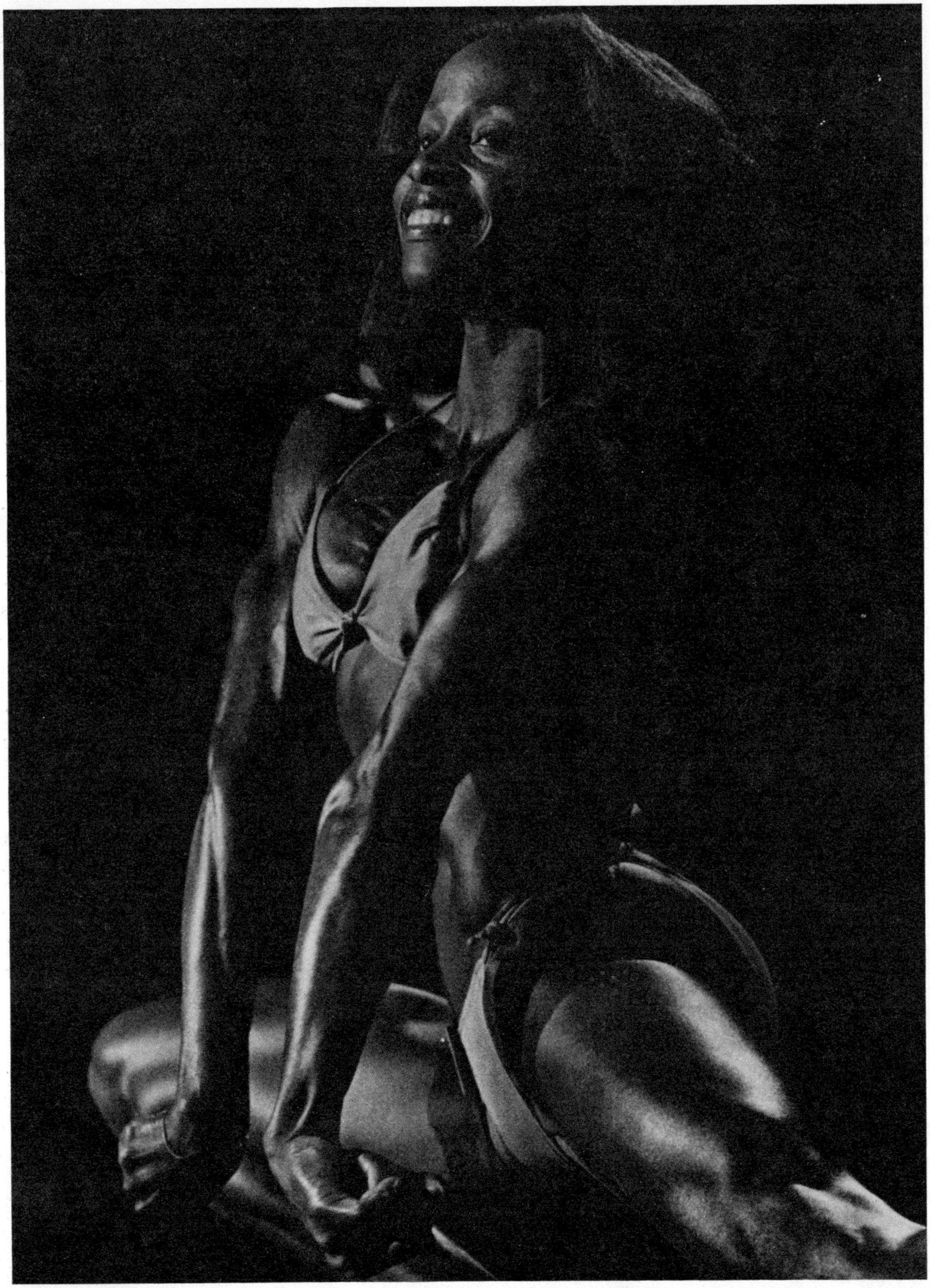

The most titled woman in bodybuilding, Carla Dunlap, displays remarkable chest development. The striations on her pectoral cleavage are rarely seen on any but the most advanced women bodybuilders.

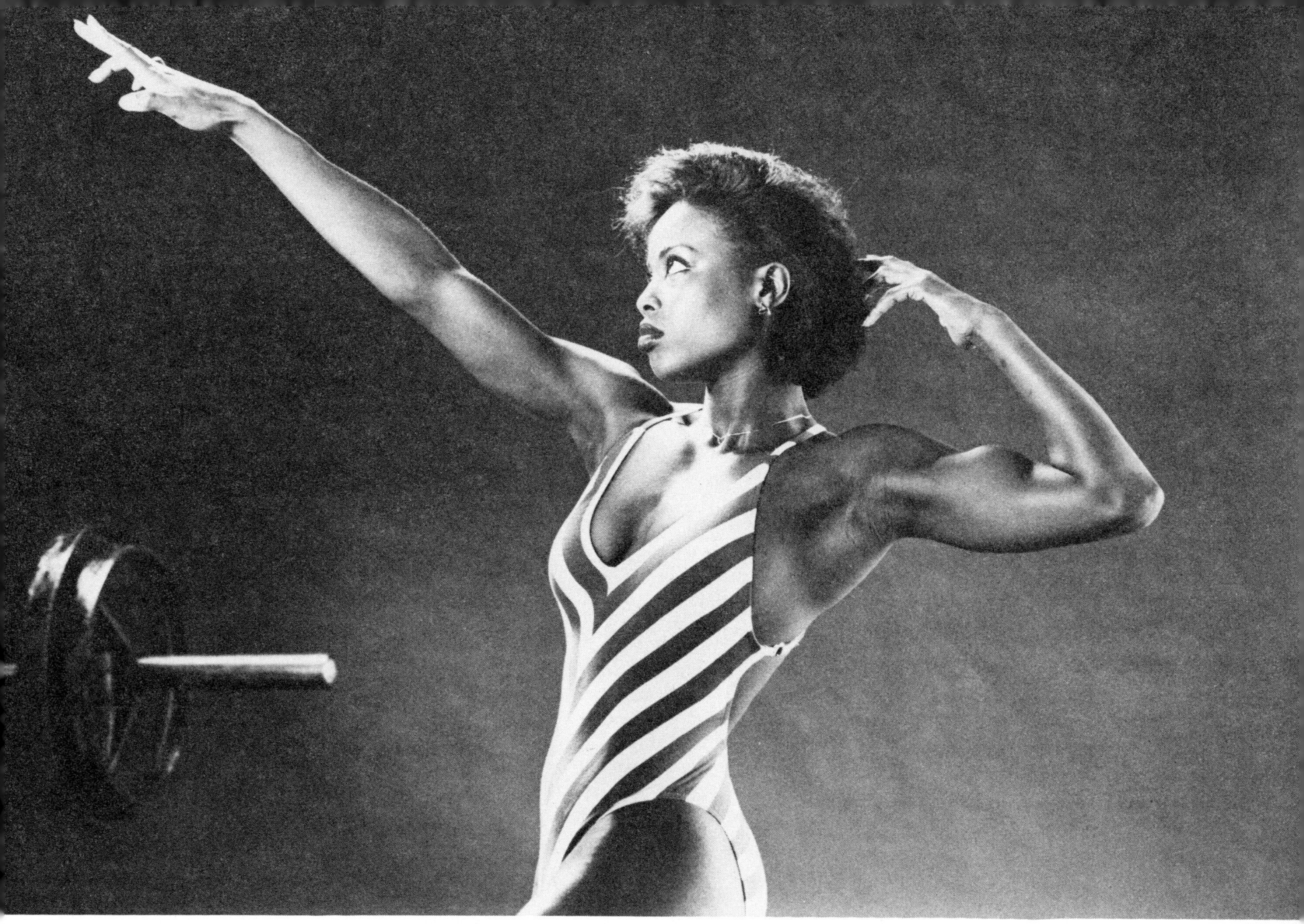

Bodybuilding champion Patsy Chapman shows off the graceful lines that weight training gives to a woman's physique. For women, training the chest can help lift the breasts and also give a fuller appearance to the bust.

should make up the bulk of your routines. Once you have a base, more isolation work can be done.

Focus on developing the torso as a whole, which includes the chest, shoulders, rib cage and triceps. Each of these areas will be trained thoroughly with basic foundation chest training. Set the foundation strongly and the gains will last for years.

Rachel McLish, Deborah Diana and Candy Csencsits are the Frank Zanes of women's bodybuilding. They have shape and symmetry, and size is secondary to proportion. This is not to imply that the women bodybuilders do not train as hard or are in any way inferior to the Carlas and Tinas of bodybuilding. The ideal chest, legs, back, and so on, will always be a matter of subjective opinion, clouded by the whims of fashion and politics.

Each type of pectoral development can be considered ideal if it fulfills all the requirements that you desire. If you like what you see, go for it!

TWO: ASSESSING YOUR CONDITION

Before you can decide what type of training program to use, you have to know your strengths and weaknesses. The more honestly you assess your pectorals, rib cage and general chest condition, the less time you lose from improper training. You can easily waste a lot of time being on a program that is too advanced, too easy, or one that doesn't meet specific goals.

The simplest way to determine what work your chest needs is to look at it in front of a full-length mirror; preferably, do this in privacy so you can relax. It's hard to get used to staring at yourself in the mirror, even for seasoned competitive bodybuilders. Arnold Schwarzenegger has said that when he looked in the mirror, he removed himself from the picture, focusing on his body as an inanimate object.

Schwarzenegger knew that to accurately assess the condition of his body, he had to let go of his ego. He could look much more objectively this way, noticing flaws he would not have caught had he been identifying with the person in the mirror. Disassociate yourself temporarily from your image so you can see what is really there.

Most people, even as their bodies change drastically in size and shape, have a hard time seeing changes or improvements. They may constantly visualize their old body image and project it onto the mirror. Visualizing this way recreates the body they'd rather not have by constantly reinforcing the old image. Successful bodybuilders see the image they want when they look in the mirror. They have a pattern for the perfect body mapped out in their minds; when they look in the mirror they project this perfect image over their imperfect body. This way they know what's needed to create the body of their dreams. To build the body of your dreams you must first create the image.

When you stand in front of the mirror, take note of posture, muscle development, size of the chest and rib cage and your bone structure. Are you an ectomorph, mesomorph or endomorph? Ectomorphs have narrow wrists, small bones and angular physiques. The typical thin marathoner is an ectomorph. The mesomorph is the naturally muscular athletic type. His shoulders are wide, hips narrow and the body lean. The endomorph is rounder-looking with narrow shoulders and a wide pelvic area. The body is soft in appearance because of an abundant supply of fat.

Ectomorphs have a hard time gaining mass and are nearly always lean. Endomorphs gain muscle mass easily but put on fat just as easily. Mesomorphs are the favored children of bodybuilding, able to grow and stay lean at the same time.

Now, take a detailed look at your chest. Is the muscle tone good and fat-free? Are the lower pecs flabby and loose? Does the muscle have good tone and definition? Is there enough size?

What type of muscle control do you have? Can you flex the muscle at will? How strong can you contract the pecs by themselves? Do you feel the muscle when you flex it, or is it slightly numb and hard to "feel"?

Look at the shape of the muscle. Are your pecs round and firm or flat? Does the upper section balance with the lower? Does the chest look powerful or does it look like a strong gust of wind could lift you off your feet? How flexible is the area? How far can you bring your arms back behind your body? Can you bring your arms straight overhead? How far can you raise your arms without arching in the lower back?

Lastly, does the chest have symmetry? Do the pecs flow into the shoulders and abdominals, or do the pecs look out of place and overdeveloped compared to the rest of

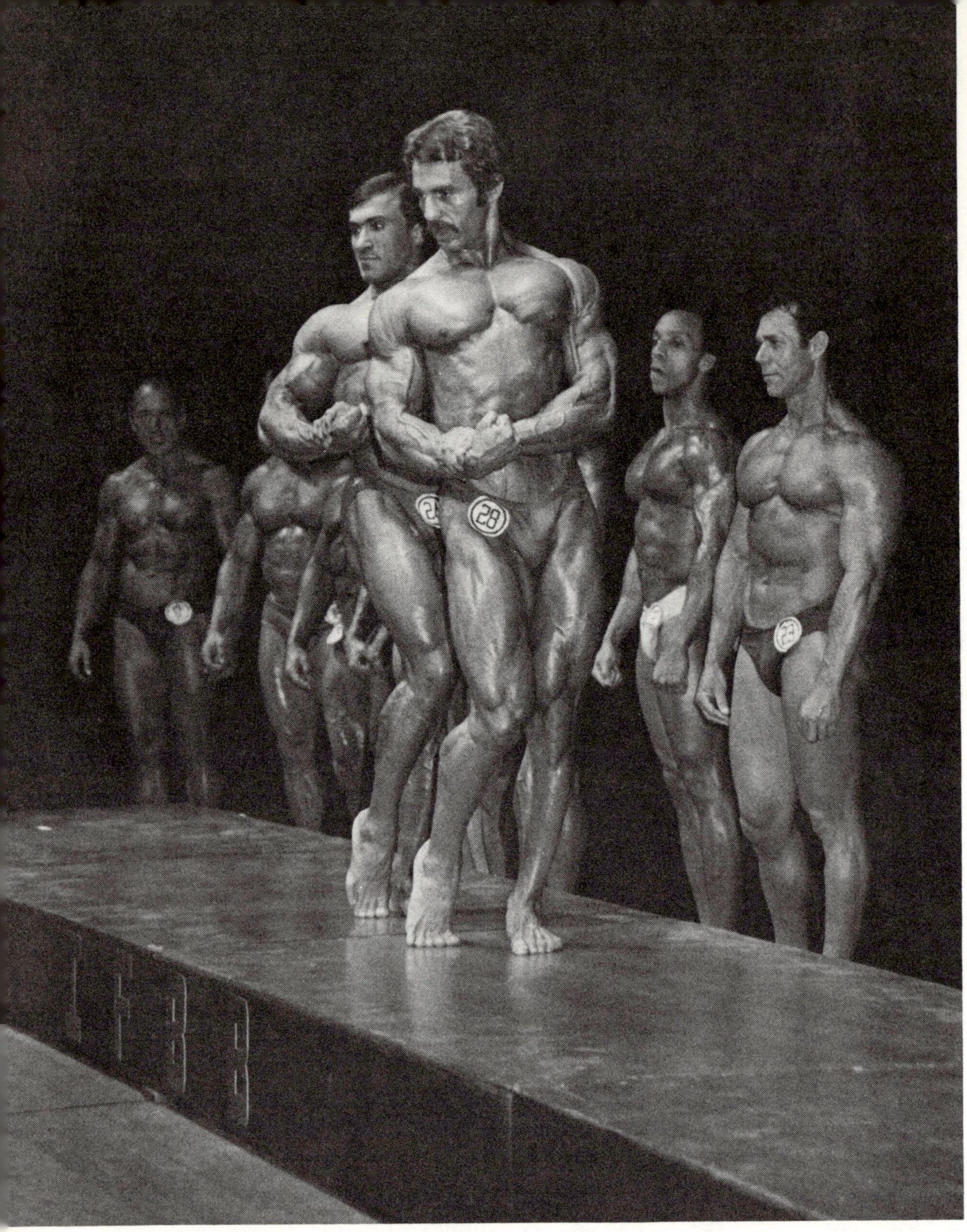

In this professional men's lineup the competitors hit a side chest pose for the judges. This pose is used primarily to display depth in the chest.

the physique? Perhaps they're small enough to warrant specialized chest training.

Consider all of these questions before deciding on the type of program you need. Again, the more honestly and accurately you assess the condition of your chest, the easier it will be to make radical changes. Here is a breakdown of the most important chest characteristics to assess and what good condition will consist of.

Size. If your chest doesn't have a modicum of size (hypertrophy of muscle fibers), you will have difficulty getting any other type of chest condition. For example, if you don't have enough muscle tissue, definition is not going to be seen and the same is true with strength or muscle density. If enough muscle mass hasn't been built up, none of these conditions will develop. For the beginner, size is a priority. My students always train for strength and size with a variety of rep schemes and basic compound exercises before specializing in any type of refinement program. You must lay a foundation before you try to build a house.

Shape. Although size is a key focus point, especially for beginners, the shape of the muscle is affected by the exercises you choose, and, more significantly, how you do those exercises. With a basic exercise like the Bench Press, you can alter performance (changing the angle slightly, for example) so radically that the same muscle groups are not affected. Look carefully at the shape of your chest area and pick the proper exercise based on your priorities. Shaping exercises isolate the specific muscle you desire. This takes a very strong program, such as flyes with dumbbells or cable, pec dec, cable crossovers and variations of basic exercises including the Neck Bench Press or very wide-grip benches.

Symmetry. Technically, symmetry is how one side of the body relates to the other in size and shape. For bodybuilders it means how the shape, definition and size of the muscles flow together and create an overall appearance. Balance is the key word when speaking of symmetry. If one aspect of the chest is underdeveloped or overdeveloped, the muscle is lacking in symmetry. Of course, good symmetry is highly subjective.

Strength. Does your chest have pushing power? If you train it for strength, that is exactly what you will get. The chest muscles work best in concert with the other upper torso muscles, such as the shoulders, triceps, and even the lats. If pressing movements such as the Bench Press, Dips or overhead presses give you problems, a strength program will help immensely. Training for strength is almost like size-training, with the emphasis on basic compound exercises, low reps and explosive movements. Strength training is also, as definition training, very rewarding. Seeing the pounds go up and the extra plates go on the bar gives immediate gratification and feedback. Strength training, unlike bodybuilding, is very straightforward. Either you can lift a certain amount of weight for a certain amount of reps or you can't. There is nothing subjective about it. Given the highly subjective nature of the rest of the bodybuilding world, this can be a refreshing and satisfying way to train with weights.

Muscle thickness or density. A chest can look big and yet not have the hardness and muscle density vital to a completely developed chest. Is your chest hard and muscular even while you stand relaxed? As we discussed before, the type of training you do has a major effect on how the chest looks even while standing relaxed. Muscle density usually is apparent when the muscle groups appear thick and hard and look like they're carved from hardwood or chiseled from stone.

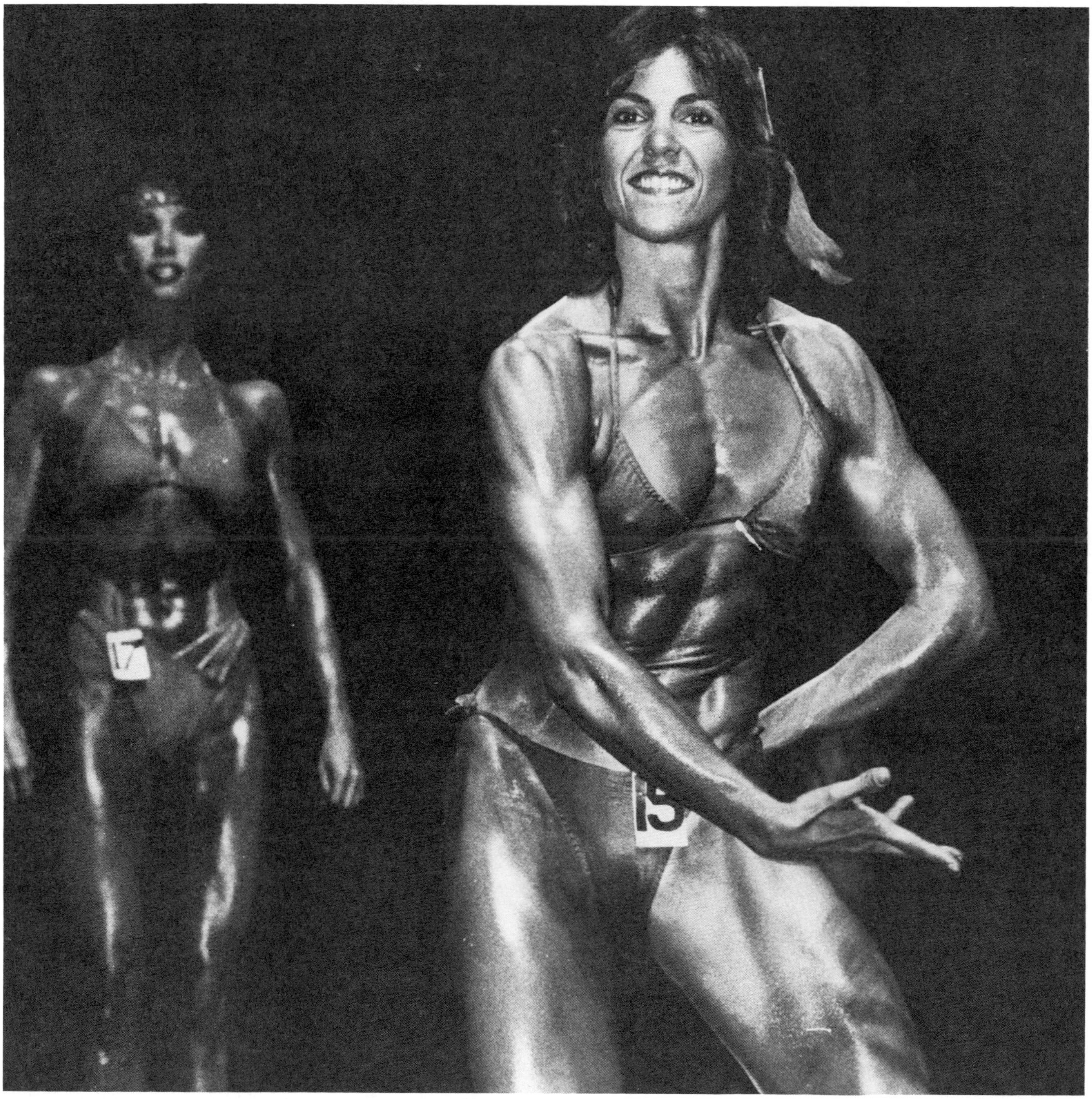

Bodybuilding and powerlifting women's champion, Agi Balogh, attributes much of her impressive upper-body development and strength to her early emphasis on the Bench Press.

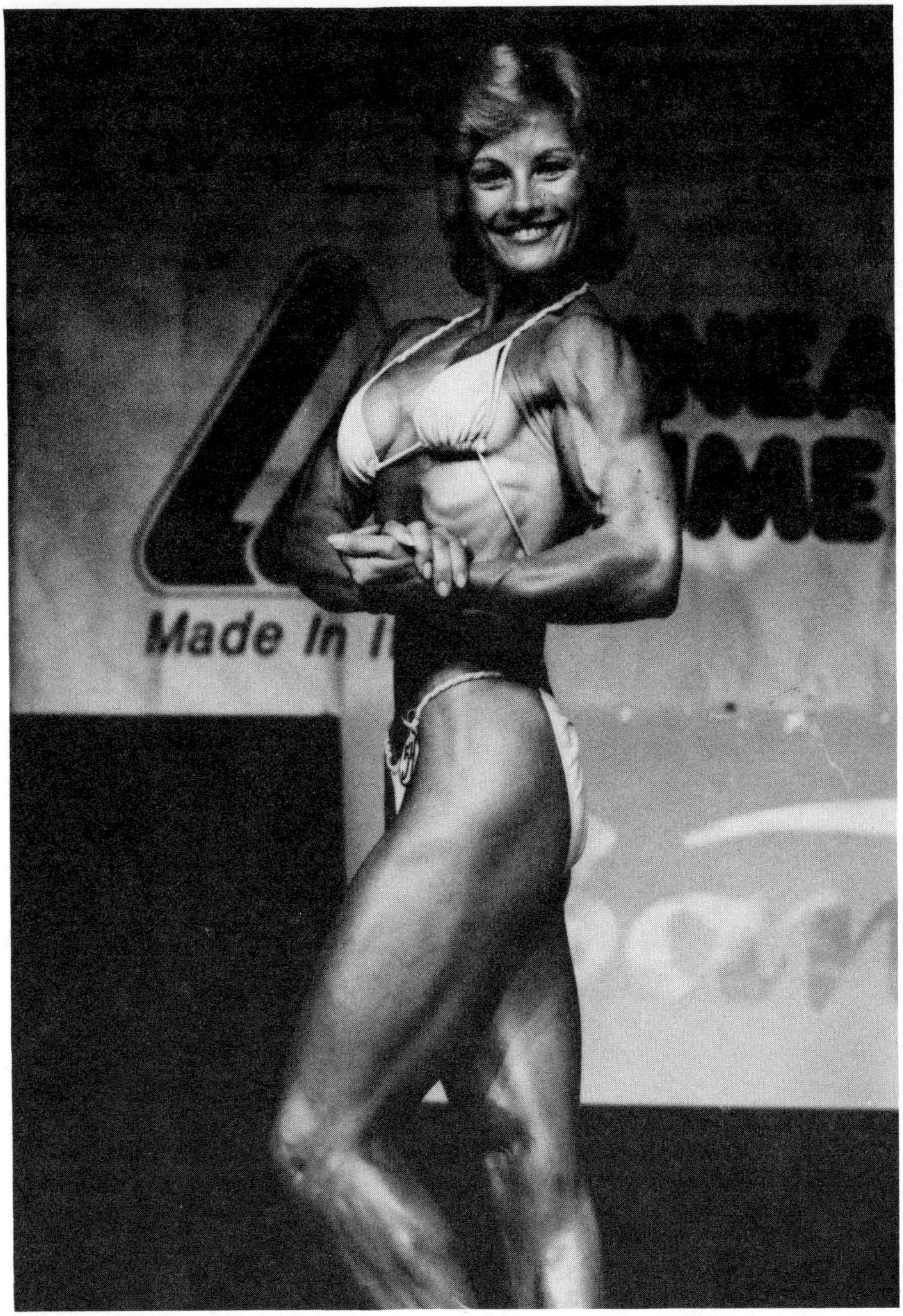

1984 USA Women's Bodybuilding Championships winner, Velma Buckles, shows off her chest, arm and shoulder development in this side chest pose.

The dense muscle comes from very heavy and hard training and doesn't result from endurance or lighter, high-rep training. This is not to say one is good and the other bad, but usually thick chest muscles have been subjected to a higher workload. Size and thickness often go together, as the two types of training are similar. You can, however, increase the size of the muscle without increasing the thickness by training the capillary and endurance systems of the chest more than the basic fibers.

Rib cage. Without a solidly built, strong rib cage, the pectoral muscles will always appear flat and unimpressive. The rib cage is the mantle upon which your prize pecs will rest, so it must be of the same high caliber as the pecs. Rib cage specialization programs stimulate growth from the inside out by alternating heavy breathing exercises (such as breathing squats) with stretching exercises (such as Straight Arm Pullovers). Rib cage specialization opens as well as builds the entire rib cage and torso area.

Skin tone. The skin is not usually covered in a chapter on training, but I firmly believe training correctly improves skin tone as well as muscle tone. If you plan to compete in bodybuilding, it is essential to maintain beautiful skin, because it is always taken into account by the judges. The winners almost always have healthy, glowing skin. Sweating is very important for healthy skin, which is one reason why saunas are popular after a hard workout.

If your skin is pale and pasty, getting into a safe sun tanning program will be well worth the time and investment. Tanned skin will make you look harder and more muscular, and the sweating that results from sun tanning will help cleanse the skin.

CHOOSING A TRAINING PROGRAM

After you assess the shape of your pecs and upper torso, you will need to choose a training program that best suits your needs. As with evaluating your chest, you must be objective and emotionally removed from choosing the appropriate workout schedule. What you need is a treasure map to your goals. Every technique in bodybuilding training stresses an individual mechanism; the response you get is totally determined by the mechanism you overload. That is why it is imperative to know how to stimulate each cellular system so you can prioritize workouts and be efficient.

Common sense will tell you that if you train with light weight, high repetitions and fairly low intensity (activity that can be continued for long periods of time), the result won't be massive strength and power.

In bodybuilding, you must ask your muscles to do a very specific task that they have not attempted or accomplished before, in order to start the depletion/adaptation process. Asking your body to work at levels far and above what it has ever done before is not necessary. You need just enough overload to stimulate the muscles.

The best way to achieve ideal training is to have a progressive mentality. Powerlifters are always thinking about putting more weight on the bar. They work at dispelling their fear of heavy weight. When they increase their weights, though, they add just enough to surpass their previous limit, knowing this ensures future gains. Consistent big jumps will burn you out. Robert Kennedy, publisher of *Muscle Mag International*, believes you should always leave a little extra for the next workout, and so does two-time Mr. Universe Bill Pearl, who trains hard but not to exhaustion.

There are many factors to consider before deciding the appropriate program. What is your goal: Size? Strength? Both? How much time do you have to train? How much time out of the gym do you want to devote? How quickly do you want to achieve your dream chest? Both long- and short-term goals are very important.

In short, how committed to achieving physique goals are you? This is a major consideration: The stronger your motivation, the easier it will be to train to your limit and become more disciplined. Your current condition and how hard you want to work will determine the program you choose. If you're a beginner but already committed to chest perfection, take your time and do it right. Skipping through levels too quickly won't bring good results. Enjoy where you are now and get to know your body.

The training facility you use will have some bearing on what programs you can follow; however, professional gyms with all the equipment are becoming more widespread.

Let's consider the more important factors that will determine which program you choose.

How Much Time Do You Have?

The amount of time you can invest in training will have a lot to do with what program you can follow. Remember, the longer and harder you train the more recovery time you need. If you are a busy executive who works long hours under pressure, a program requiring high volume and heavy workloads is not going to be suitable. High training volume and workloads are equivalent to having a high-stress job.

Diminishing Returns

In the beginning there are easy gains. As you become stronger, improvements come much more slowly. At intermediate and advanced-intermediate levels you need to do some unique training to continue improving. You can't train a lot harder, because you'll risk injury and mental burnout. When you finally see gains after a plateau, you'll know it immediately. The muscle you're working will be sore but stronger. It will stay pumped for hours.

When you reach the point of diminishing returns in chest training, you must deplete and then fully recover to stimulate growth. This process is part of the art and mastery of natural bodybuilding (without drugs).

As a trainer, it's hard to understand why so many people put up with minor gains when they're working hard. When I work hard I want results. You should consider the training program as the reason for slow progress. It you think it's the source of your lack of gains, get a new program. Considering how the body works, changing a routine can "shock" the body into a new growth cycle.

The body works in cycles or biorhythms, the waves in the ocean of life. Although there will be down cycles, committed bodybuilders will work through them to get the most out of their training. Your strength level fluctuates daily.

Scott Wilson, Mr. International winner and a man with common sense, believes that listening to your body is the key. "Some days I can go in the gym and squat with 500 pounds for 10 reps, but sometimes I go in there and can't do a single rep with that weight. 'What's it all about,' I'd ask myself? The body isn't to blame, it's the mind. The strength is there but for some reason you can't tap into it. You can't get motivated. The key is to work to your maximum, because it's going to be changing a lot. Always go to the limit and keep training your mind."

Once you realize everyone has ups and downs while training, you can learn to listen to your body. You'll find out how hard you should work out, what food to eat and how long you need for recovery. The stronger your mental control, the easier it is to cancel negative attitudes and train through the minor down cycles.

Muscle Specificity

Here's an acronym you should remember for better training results—S.A.I.D., or Specific Adaptation to Imposed Demands. The goal is to get the body to adapt only to the specific type of stress you apply. Don't expect big, dense muscles if you only lift light weights that don't challenge you. If your muscles aren't challenged, they will not respond. And if you train them for strength, don't expect endurance!

Training comes down to realizing your strengths and weaknesses and training them accordingly.

Determining stresses for specific adaptation is simple. For strength training, low reps, high intensity (85 to 95 percent max weight) and low total volume (two to four sets) do the job best. For localized muscle endurance, use lighter loads with 40 to 50 percent of maximum effort and 30 to 40 reps per set. Power training also requires light loads (about 50 percent) so speed can be practiced. You cannot move heavy weights fast. Being explosive with a heavy weight is a necessity, but when using close to maximum weight, you can expect a slow lift. To train for speed, you must practice with loads that can be done fast.

Your Athletic Background

Regardless of your athletic background or current shape, if you're a beginning bodybuilder you should do foundation training for one year. Even three-time Mr. Olympia Frank Zane begins his yearly training cycle as a beginner. You will be doing basic exercises with higher reps and lower intensity; focus on form and finding your limit. Concentrate on getting the proper angle, form, resistance and "feel" to each exercise.

The more "muscular" your training history, the easier bodybuilding will be for you. Gymnastics, martial arts, football and wrestling are excellent for preparing your muscles for the stresses of bodybuilding.

Endurance athletes, although usually not as muscular, seem to adapt well to bodybuilding. I have coached many endurance athletes (including Olympic speedskater Eric Heiden and national-class cyclists Keith Vierra and Sterling McBride) and I'm amazed by what they can take.

Heiden in particular was impressive. He has trained with weights many years (he has done 100 reps with almost 300 pounds in the Squat!), and his concentration and focus was as intense as anything I've seen. Once he began an exercise, he took it to the end, no matter how painful.

Present Training Program

Once you have assessed your condition and determined the program you need, you'll probably want to modify your existing program. Most people need to totally revamp their program, especially if they have been on the same one for more than two months. A total change of exercises, sets, reps and training tempo will do the job. Remember, though, always train your least-liked exercises as if they were your favorite.

Cross Training

Cross training, or training simultaneously in different disciplines, was popularized by triathletes who, because of the nature of their event, need to exercise in three different disciplines—swimming, cycling and running. Cross training can also apply to bodybuilding. In its simplest form, you would weight train one day and do alternate forms of exercise on other days.

Cross training is nothing new, though. Decathletes (who compete in 10 track and field events) and other multi-sport athletes have been cross training for years.

Training for maximum adaptation in strength, coordination, speed and endurance without overtraining can be very tricky, especially if you are a runner or an athlete who primarily uses one body part. Training the primary muscles for endurance and strength without overworking requires understanding how to vary intensity and knowing when you should not train.

You must constantly listen to the signals your body is sending and alter the schedule when you think you need a rest. Recovery always precedes adaptation; if you have not fully recovered, you're risking injury and illness.

I will stress this throughout the book: Overtraining is the beginning of the end. There must be easy days so that your hard efforts can be genuinely hard. Without rest, you cannot be intense. Conversely, if you never train intensely, it will be difficult to take days off because you haven't experienced the true fatigue of intense training. It is no big deal to take a day off if you are training to your limit. Indeed, if you never feel like taking days off to rest, you probably aren't training intensely.

The athlete who trains without drugs that enhance recuperation must be a master of reading the body. If his routine says to go heavy and he's feeling depleted, he'll risk injury by training through the fatigue. Of course, if he sets up his program correctly, he shouldn't be depleted on a day that calls for intense training.

Proper scheduling is the best way to achieve maximum adaptation with the least risk of overtraining. Prioritize your workouts. Do the most important exercises and weakest body parts at the beginning of your workout or training cycle.

THREE: RIB CAGE TRAINING

You would never think of building a house's foundation in the sand, because it would quickly break apart and collapse. Yet many bodybuilders train their chests without taking the time to build the foundation on which the entire torso rests—the rib cage.

Rib cage training is essential to the beginning bodybuilder, or even the intermediate or advanced bodybuilder who was never properly instructed in foundation and strength building. Foundation training should take place before isolation-style bodybuilding.

For those whose main goal is building size in the entire body or just the chest area, it makes sense to spend from three to five months on rib cage specialization before beginning routines designed to build primarily the pectoral muscles. Pectoral muscles built on a small rib cage will always look flat and small, especially when doing the side chest pose and other poses designed to enhance the rib cage and pec area.

Bodybuilders such as Arnold Schwarzenegger, Casey Viator and Roy Callender have incredible rib cages. As we mentioned in Chapter 1, Schwarzenegger was so huge that you could come in from the rain if you stood close enough! When Schwarzenegger did the side chest pose, almost no one could stand next to him. His 60-inch chest was the cornerstone of his physique, giving him a huge advantage in physique competition. When he stood sideways he was almost as deep as two bodybuilders put together!

Most beginning programs work the rib cage because they are based on multi-joint compound exercises such as the Bench Press, Squat and Pullover. When the rib cage is stretched (as in Pullovers) or forced to expand (during heavy squat work) the effect is dramatic, especially when the stretching is done immediately after the heavy breathing exercise. By concentrating on the rib cage expansion during Squats, Pullovers, Bench Presses and Dips, muscularity and strength of the rib cage can be enhanced.

Connecting the mind and muscles is essential. You must be able to "feel" the stretch and the contractions in order to get the most from them. Beginners are astounded that they are supposed to feel the exercises from start to finish. Most beginners assume that as long as they are moving the weights and huffing and puffing, they will get results. If only that were true!

As discussed in Chapter 1, the rib cage is connected to the sternum by cartilage, which, when we are young and still growing, is capable of stretching and expanding. Heavy breathing work and stretching can cause big increases in rib cage size in adolescents.

Even if the rib cage itself doesn't grow to accommodate the stress, the muscles surrounding the cage will grow larger, stronger and thicker from consistent rib cage work. If the rib cage doesn't grow larger, but it looks that way, does it matter?

When you're on the beach, it doesn't matter. If it looks good there (or on the posing dias) and the impression of size is obvious, the measurement shouldn't matter. Much of the controversy over bodybuilders just "looking big" and not really being strong originated with pump-style training. This type of training "plumps" up the mitochondria and capillary systems and size increases occur without strength increases. For modern-day bodybuilding, though, no one is that interested in the actual measurements.

Nothing sets off a physique like the muscularity surrounding the rib cage and upper abdominal area

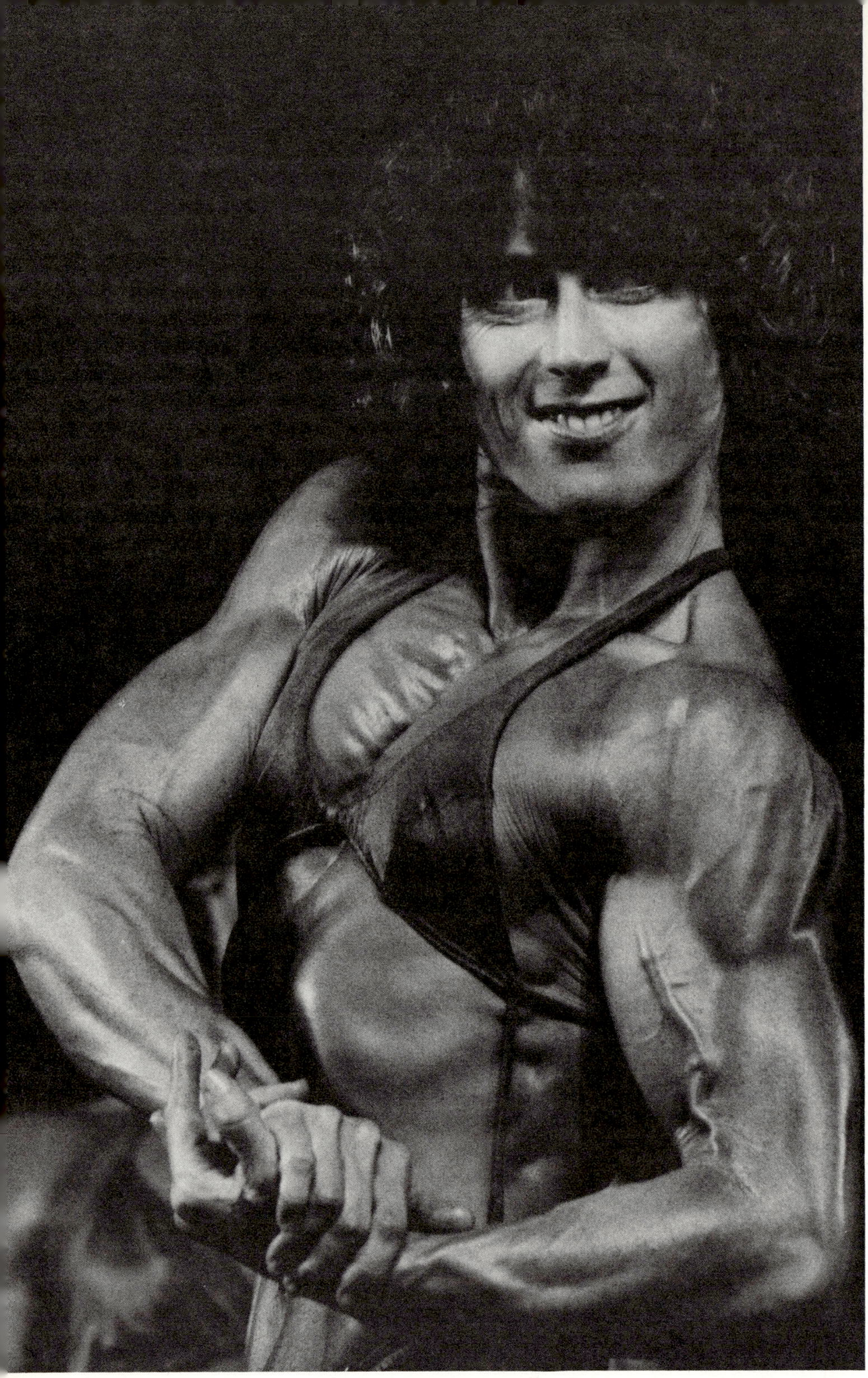

When it comes to muscular development on a woman, few can compare with this lady—known to fans and friends only as "Pillow." Her chest development is so advanced you can count each striation in her pecs.

(which is also built up through rib cage work). It lifts the entire torso and adds depth and thickness to the chest and surrounding areas. Carla Dunlap's muscle mass and muscularity gains in her rib cage gave her physique the centerpiece it needed, adding elegance and refinement by lifting her torso up and increasing size and muscle quality.

Why take the time for rib cage specialization? Because it will increase your lung capacity and give the internal organs more room to operate. This is very important for good health.

Heavy Squat and Pullover work can add pounds of muscle over the entire body and stimulate the metabolism to large muscle mass and/or body weight gains. Old-time bodybuilders were into this routine when they wanted serious weight gains—heavy, high-rep breathing exercises that turned the metabolism anabolic and built size from the inside out.

There are a few alternatives, however, on how to put a rib cage specialization program together. The most fundamental workout involves super-setting (doing exercises back to back with no rest) Breathing Squats and Barbell Pullovers. This is perhaps the hardest, but also the most effective method of producing a large rib cage area and muscle mass gains. All beginning bodybuilders still in their growing phase (ages 15 to 21) should spend time doing high-rep Breathing Squats and Pullovers when trying to gain weight.

The program is simple. Breathing Squats involve using a barbell no heavier than your body weight and doing high numbers of reps. The magic number usually falls between 20 and 25. The first 10 to 12 should be done continuously, breathing in before going down; hold your breath on the descent and through the first movement up from the full squat position. Then exhale strongly on the exertion through the completion of the rep where the process begins again. After rep 10 or 12 you should take four to five slow full breaths between each rep. If your body weight is so low that squatting for 10 reps is easy, add as much weight as necessary, but the last 10 reps should not be forced.

The purpose of this workout is to stimulate heavy breathing and then stretch the rib box as much as possible while the lungs expand. Sound like fun? I knew you'd like it! If you can get into high-rep Squats and Pullovers, chances are you'll love the rest of bodybuilding. As you take deep breaths, shrug your shoulders toward your ears to take the stress off the diaphragm. This allows you to take in more oxygen and expand the rib box even further. Shrugging the shoulders for the last five reps works the entire upper torso.

After finishing the squats, go to Barbell Pullovers. Lie with your shoulders across an exercise bench, face up. Using a shoulder-width grip, lower the bar with straight arms behind you in an arc. Let the finish of the stretch start the upward motion. The finish of any stretch is the beginning of the next contraction. Take advantage of this. Do not bounce the weight out of the bottom but feel where the stretch ends and use it to help you begin the contraction. Some Nautilus machines have this contraction built in. It's called a pre-stretch.

Mr. International Scott Wilson displays his massive upper body size. A deep, wide rib cage is the foundation for impressive pectoral development.

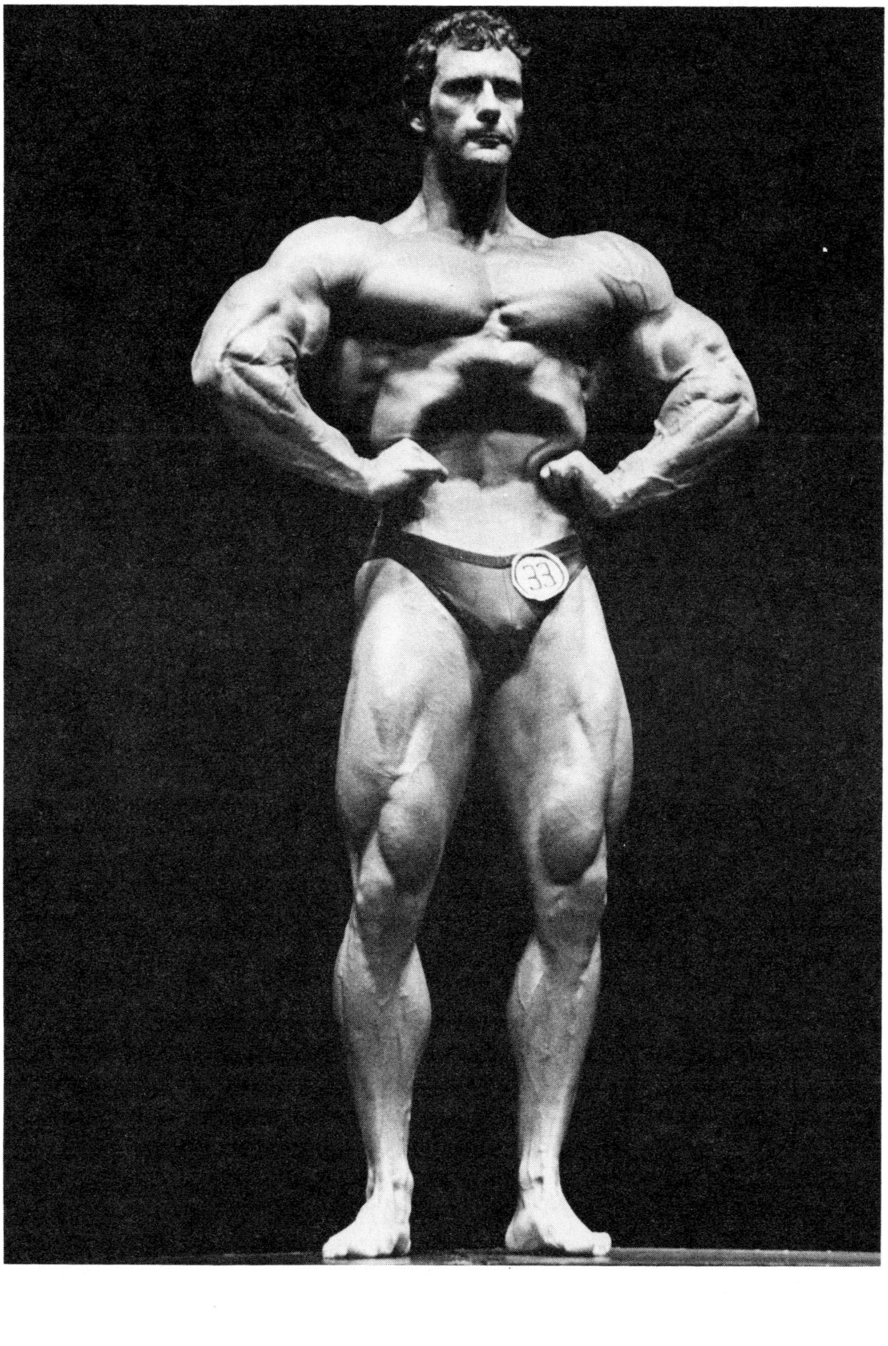

Relax the triceps as the bar lowers behind you or you cannot achieve a full stretch. Keeping the hips low is also very important for getting the full stretch. The torso should be tilted up as if something was pulling you up from the ceiling with a cord attached to your sternum. Think about your upper back (not lower) arch when you do Pullovers.

Some lifters recommend Pullovers while lying flat on the exercise bench. This is effective for stretching the rib cage, but you must use extremely light weight. Keeping the hips down helps you maintain balance when you use heavier weights. Remember, you should do 20 reps. Be careful with the straight arms, because your elbows might complain if you let the weight get too heavy. Bending the arms slightly and then locking them in the bent position works well for those with sore elbows or if you use a dumbbell.

Pullover Specialization

By changing the angle of the dumbbell (you can use dumbbells or a barbell), you can emphasize either the lats or the chest (tilt the dumbbell forward, through the tops of the fingers, for chest emphasis). Pullovers also work the serratus muscles, those fingerlike muscles under the pecs and to the sides of the abdominals. Most exercises take the muscle through one type of contraction, either a length, peak or mid-range contraction. Pullovers make the torso work hard through a length and mid-range

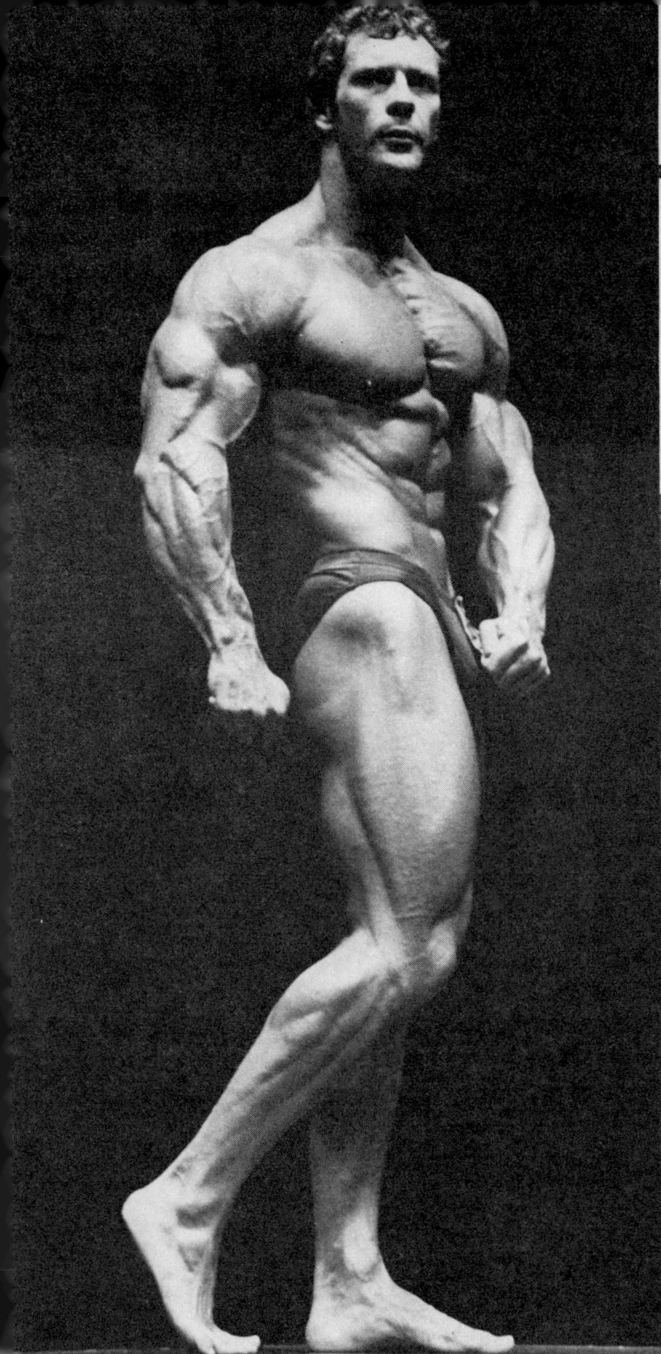

The remarkable development of professional bodybuilder Scott Wilson is the result of many years of hard, intensive training.

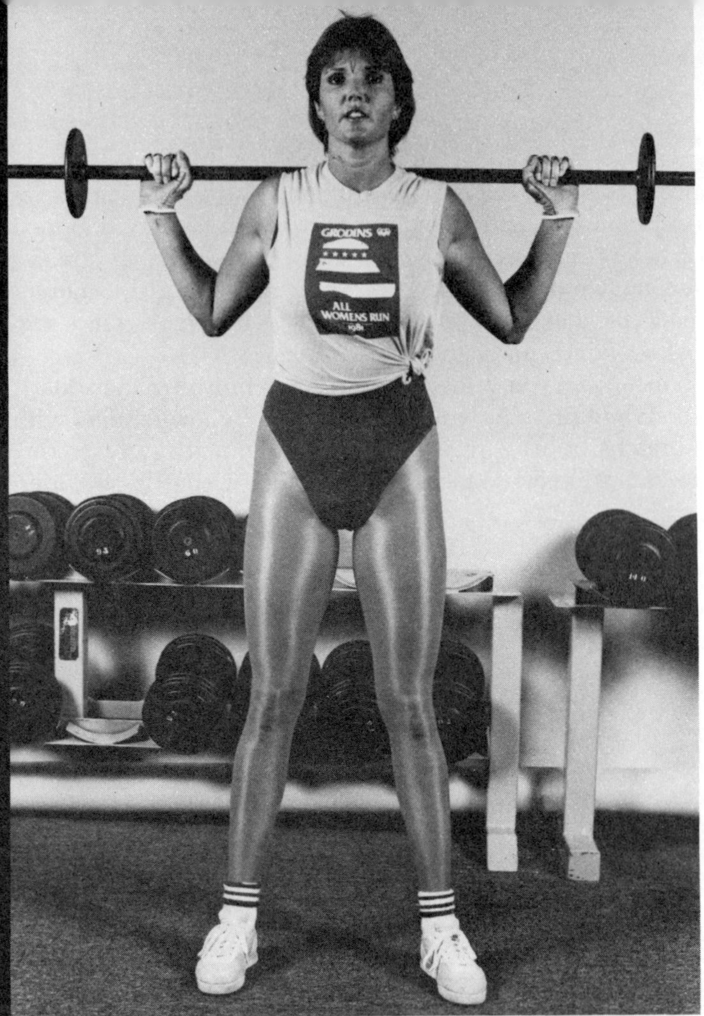

Gayle O'Donnell demonstrates the starting position for the Squat. The bar rests across your shoulders while your hands support it with a wide grip. Your toes should point slightly out and be in alignment with your knees.

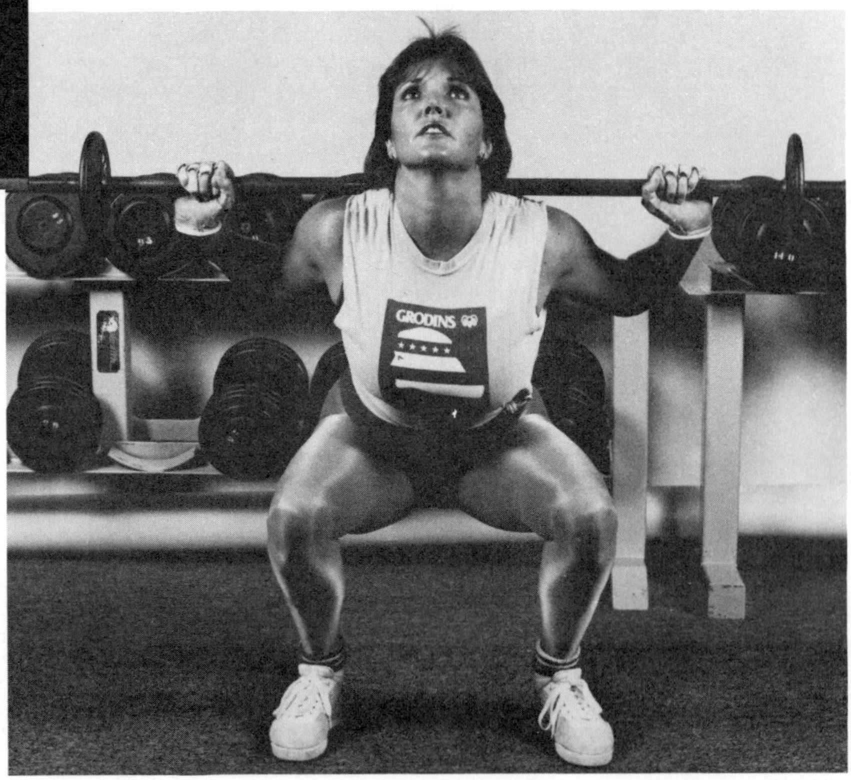

The back should be flat and head up as you descend into the Squat. At their lowest depth, the upper thighs should be perpendicular to the floor.

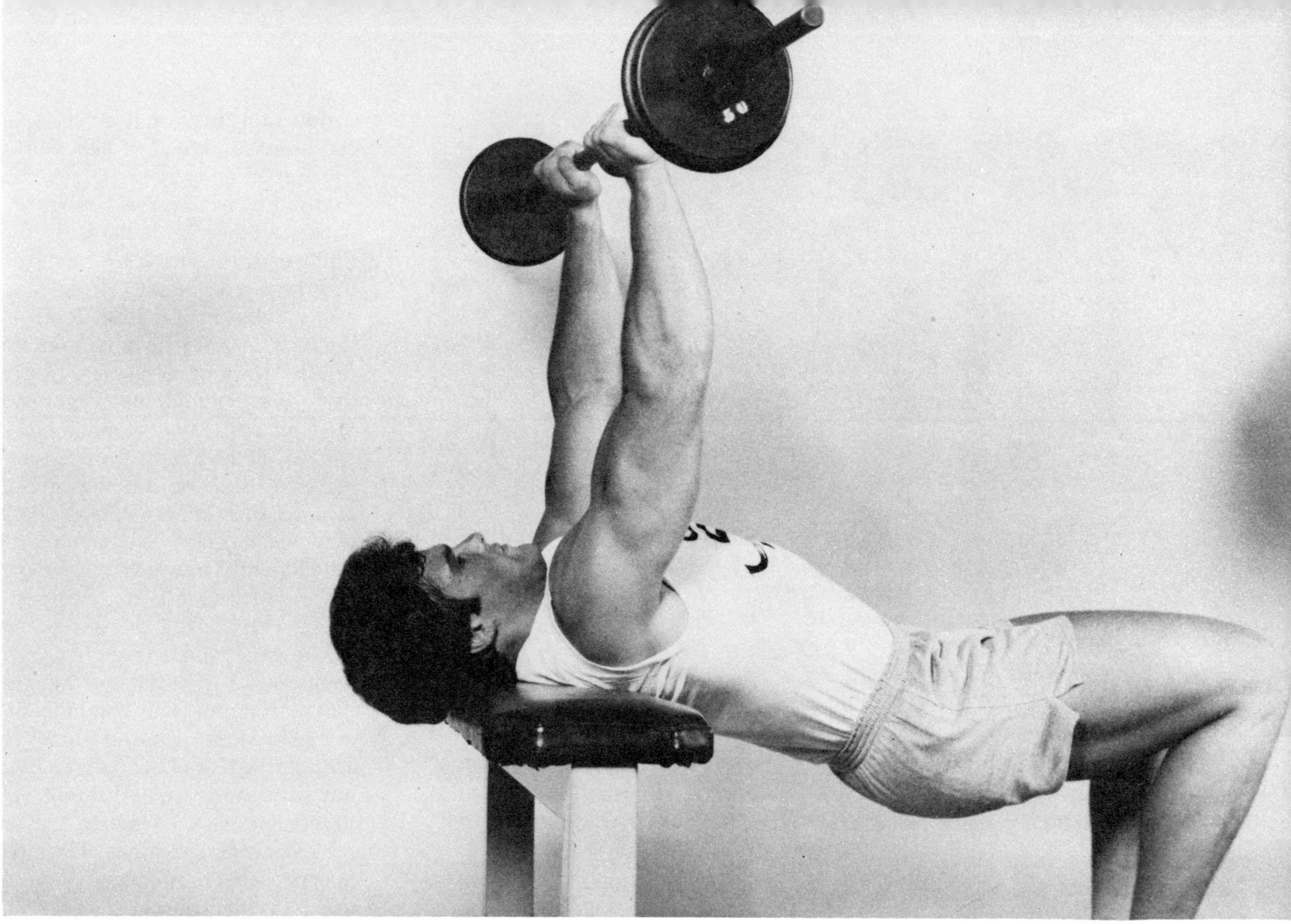

▲

The Straight Arm Pullover begins with the barbell at full arms' extension above the head. From this position you lower the barbell behind your head as far as possible.

▶

Your lungs should be full of air when you reach the maximum stretch position of a Straight Arm Pullover.

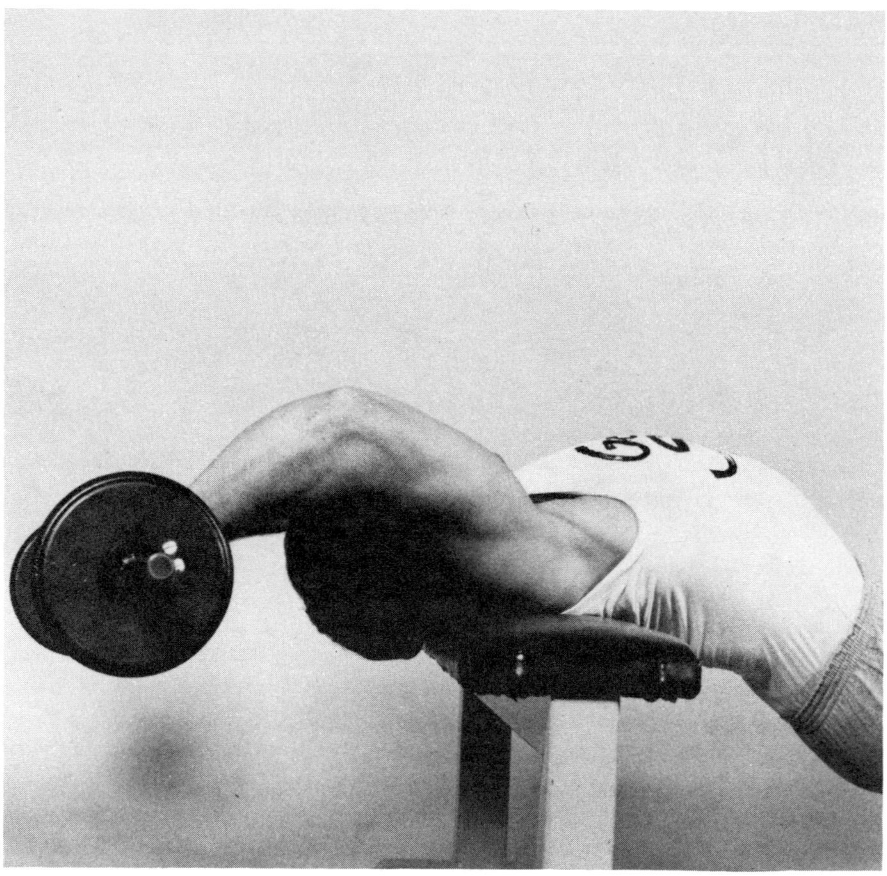

contraction, making it a very special exercise indeed. It also works the upper and inner pecs better than any other exercise. Former Mr. America Steve Michalik says "the Pullover exercise is the only true upper chest developer."

The Pullover also adds depth to the torso in a way no other exercise can. By working all the muscles of the torso simultaneously and through a full range of motion, the work of all the muscle groups is integrated. Isolation training cannot achieve this effect. When asked why his muscles did not appear bunchy and "trowled up" as most other bodybuilders' do, Schwarzenegger replied that this came from working the muscles together, with compound basic exercises and super-set training. This combination of techniques allowed him to achieve the size of the bodybuilder but with the grace and fluidity of the synchronized swimmer.

Master trainer Vince Gironda doesn't believe Pullovers do anything for the rib cage, however. Gironda feels that since the rib cage muscles are in a state of contraction while the arms are going behind the head, the muscles of the rib cage are contracting too deeply to allow expansion of the rib box. My own personal experience contradicts Gironda's findings. I believe the Pullover exercise (usually done with dumbbells and bent arms) is indispensable and has a multitude of uses for the beginning on up to the advanced bodybuilder.

Another excellent combination of exercises to deepen and thicken the rib cage is the Bench Press followed by Pullovers, or vice versa. Getting to the point of being out of breath while exercising is a very important part of increasing rib cage size or thickness. The set must be hard. Use as heavy a weight as possible with good form for high reps. Do 12 to 20 reps per set; three to four sets should be enough. Again, do this combination at the beginning of your workout, when your energy reserves are at their highest.

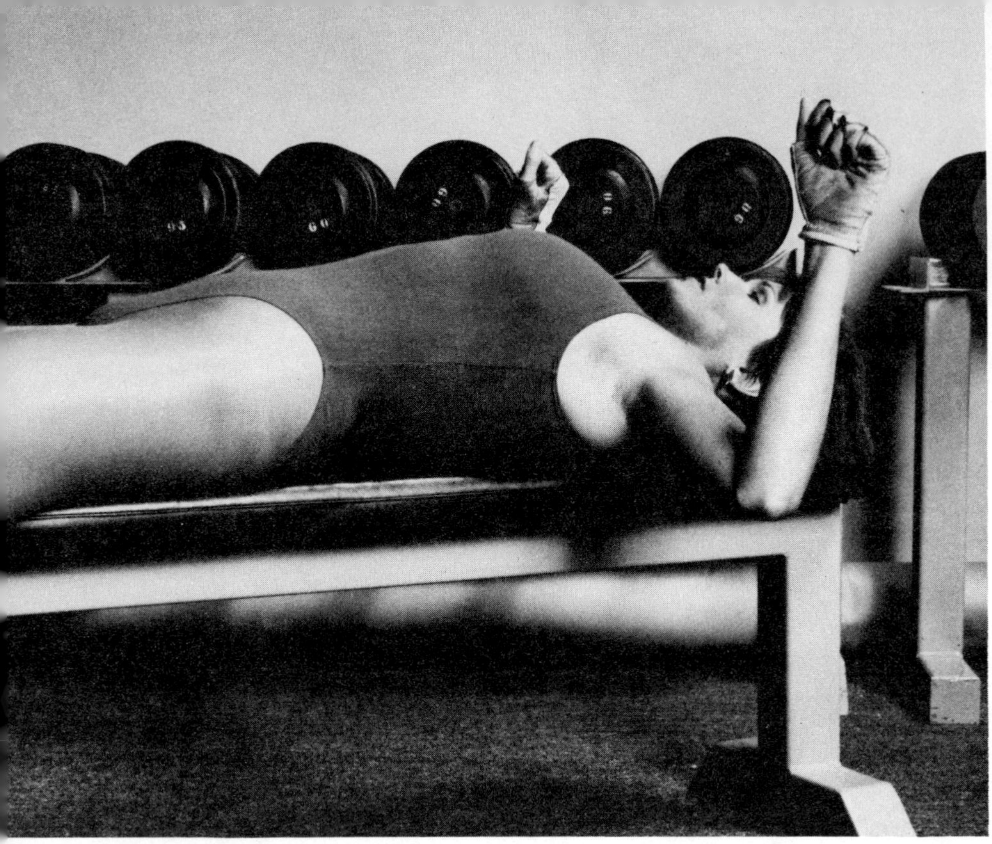

▲ *To stretch the muscles of the chest, Gayle O'Donnell goes through the motions of a Bench Press—without the bar. Lie on a narrow bench with your hands extended above you. From here pull your shoulder blades together while lifting the chest.*

▼ *This torso stretch, performed by Tami Broadfoot, is similar to a push-up, except your hips do not lift off the floor. Because the torso muscles are seldom stretched in this fashion, progress slowly at first.*

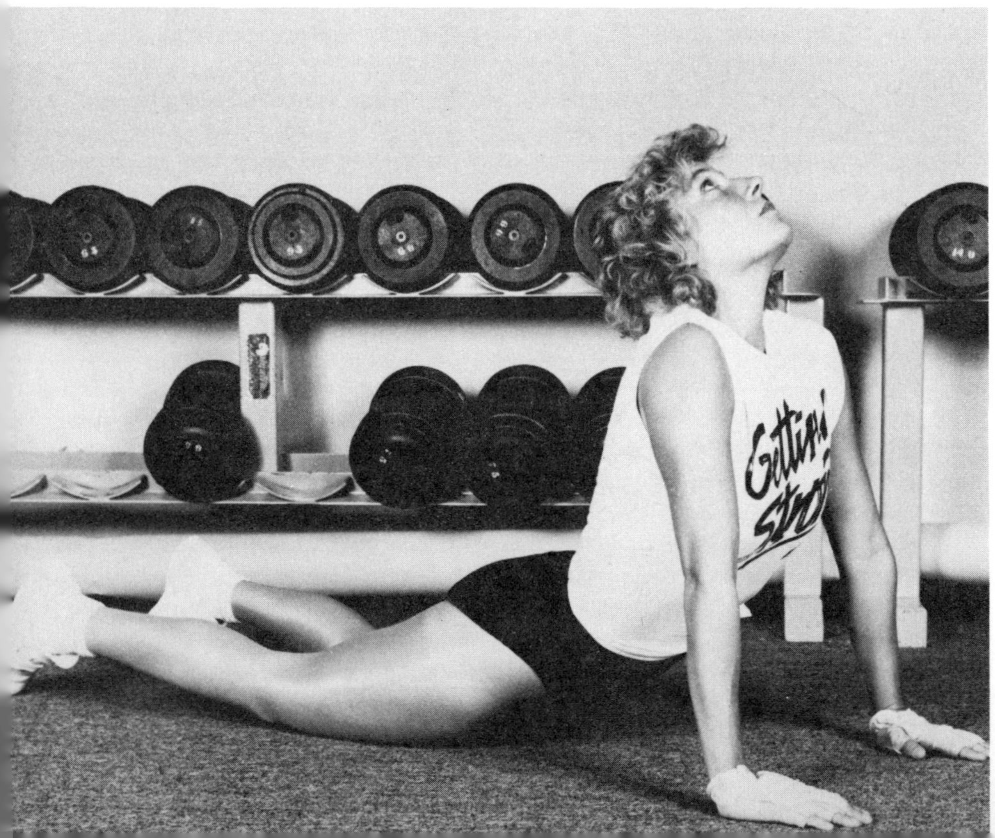

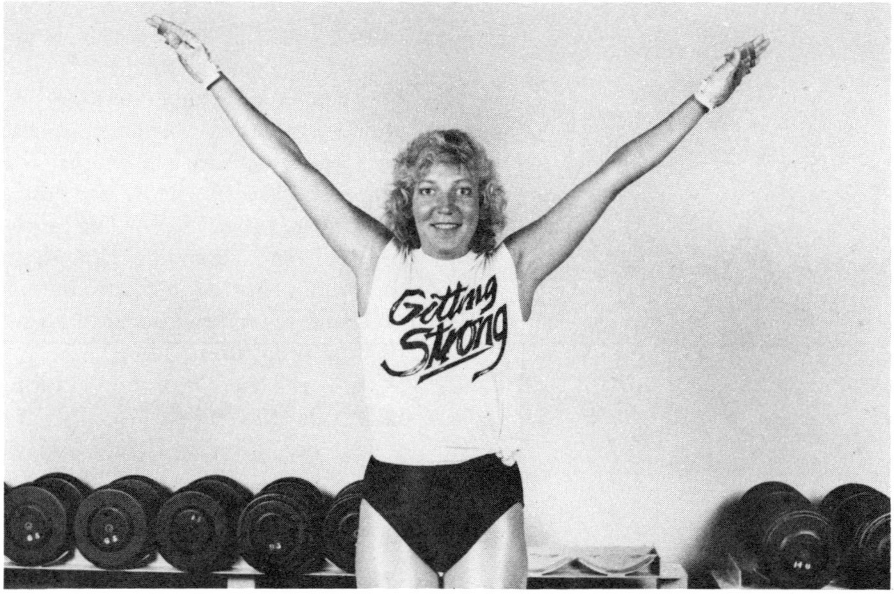

To warm up the delicate shoulder muscles, perform wide arm circles. This exercise can also be performed with light dumbbells.

This exercise increases the range of motion of the shoulders. Start by holding a stick at full arms' extension overhead, then pull it behind your back as far as possible. As your flexibility improves, move your hands closer together.

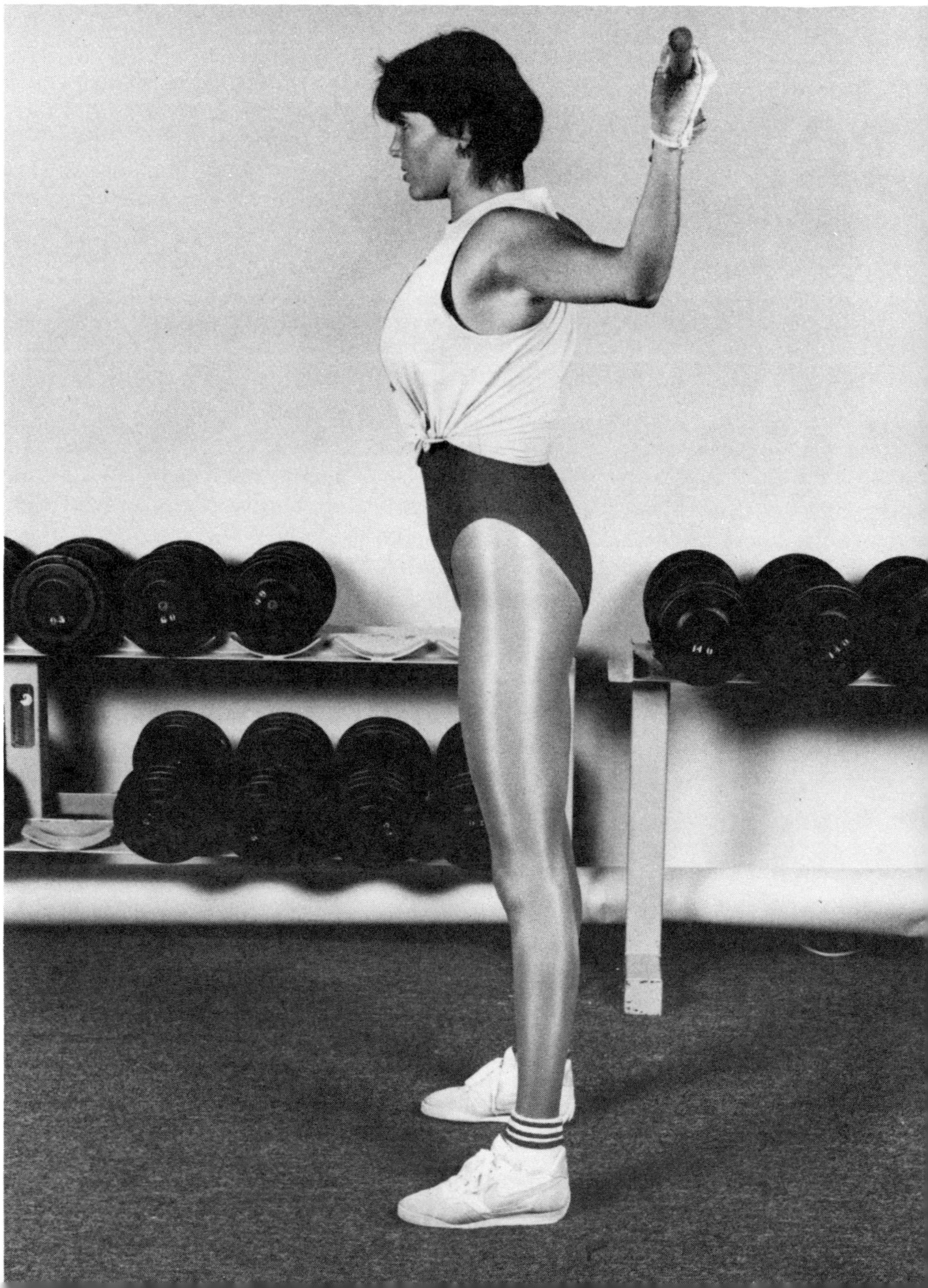

Dipping between parallel bars, with or without added weight, opens, expands and thickens not only the rib cage but the entire torso. Because of the range of motion possible with dips, considerable stress can be put on the torso using relatively light weights. You must go all the way down so that the pecs get the most stretch possible for a full contraction of the muscle groups.

Changing the position of the chest, head, elbow and back while doing dips changes the stress on the torso and hence its development. By dropping the chin onto the chest, rounding the back and keeping the elbows flared out to the sides at a 45-degree angle, the chest is isolated and worked to its maximum. The pelvis must be tucked under with the feet under the chest. The exact opposite position—head up, elbows close to the sides with feet behind you—works the triceps to the maximum.

Bench Press Specialization

Another method of increasing the rib cage size is to specialize on the Bench Press by utilizing a power bench position. The chest will be opened and lifted to meet the descending bar; it will develop flexibility and static (holding) strength. The correct position for

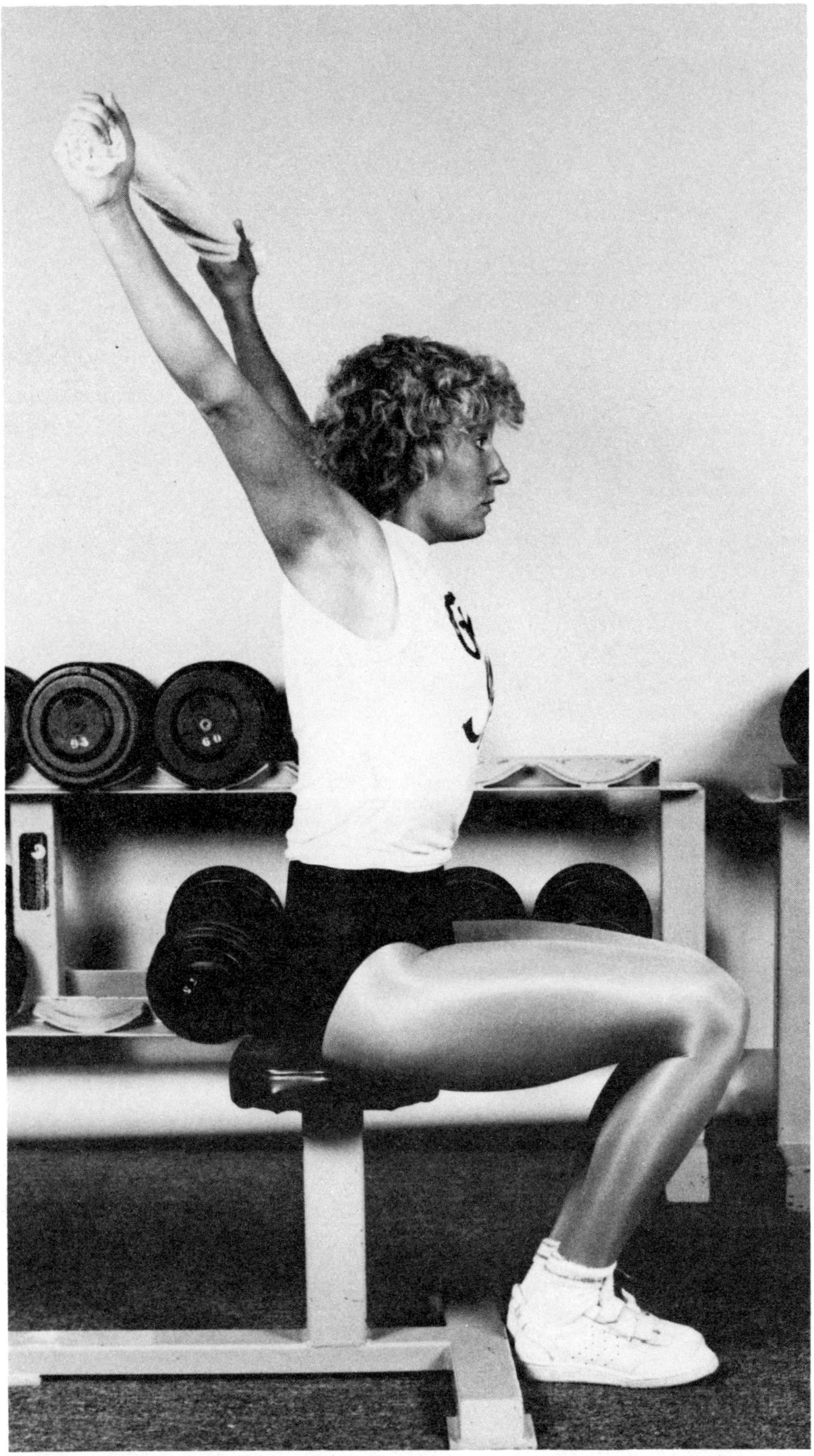

Here's another effective exercise for stretching the shoulders. While holding a towel above your head, pull the towel behind you as far as you can.

power Bench Pressing is a semi-bowed position on the bench with the chest lifted as much as possible, shoulder blades together in the back and the entire body tight. The upper back and the legs should take most of the weight. The glutes (buttocks muscles) must remain on the bench, but most of the body's weight is off them and planted on the feet and upper back.

This is the "bow" position, which is the most effective for power benching and puts a great deal of stress on the muscles of the rib cage. High reps don't work well with power benching, so keep the reps between 6 and 12 and use as heavy a weight as possible, with perfect form for three to five sets.

Flexibility

When training the chest for rib cage enlargement or for pectoral growth, upper back and shoulder flexibility is essential. Almost all of the necessary exercises for the chest and rib cage, the back included, require good flexibility.

To increase your flexibility, lie flat on your back on an exercise bench, pull the shoulder blades together as closely as possible and lift the chest up through the sternum without losing the contracted position of the shoulder blades. Hold this position for 15 seconds when you begin and work up to one minute of continuous position training. The position will teach the muscle to remember the form as well as stretch the torso.

To isolate and stretch the involved muscles even more, lie flat on your stomach on the floor and put your hands at your sides, next to your pecs. Keeping your hips as low to the ground as possible, push up to where your arms are straight, and lift your chest, head and shoulders as far up and back as possible. This helps upper back flexibility and the necessary upper back arch.

Poor range of motion in the shoulder can hinder Pullover work. Isolation stretching is the best way to improve shoulder range of motion. Before stretching the delicate shoulder area, warm up the deltoid muscles by doing arm circles with either light dumbbells or no weight at all. Move the arms in very small tight circles and expand the size of the circles as you continue, finishing with large overhead circles. Then work your way back down to small delicate circles again.

A flexible shoulder joint that is strong through its entire range of motion is much less prone to injury. In gymnastics training, before putting the joints (especially the shoulders) through high-intensity motions or contractions, we would warm up for at least an hour. We'd stretch the shoulders by using a stick and bringing it up, over and behind the head. Moving the shoulders back and forth increases the range of motion as well as any stretch. Gymnasts would always carry their own little stretching sticks and work on shoulder flexibility as often as possible. Gymnasts use the delts constantly and never take them for granted; they know the importance of stretching and warming up this area. This stretch takes practice and, like all stretching exercises, should never be forced. Avoid pain in all stretching exercises. If you can hold the stretch, you are not stretching too far.

Other methods of stretching the shoulders include reaching up overhead, grasping both hands together (if you can) and stretching the arms back behind you; don't arch the back. The stretch can be done one arm at a time, using the arm not being stretched to guide the arm being stretched back behind the head. Always keep the elbows close to the head. The longer you hold the stretch the sooner you'll see results. Stretch the shoulders from the rear by sitting upright on the floor, feet straight out in front of you; bring the arms together behind you, palms flat on the floor.

Experiment with other shoulder stretches. There are many positions and stretches for the shoulders. Bob Anderson's book, *Stretching*, is an excellent anthology of stretching movements for a myriad of sports.

This is a more advanced stretching exercise for the shoulders. Clasp both hands with your arms straight, then lift them up and behind your head as far as possible.

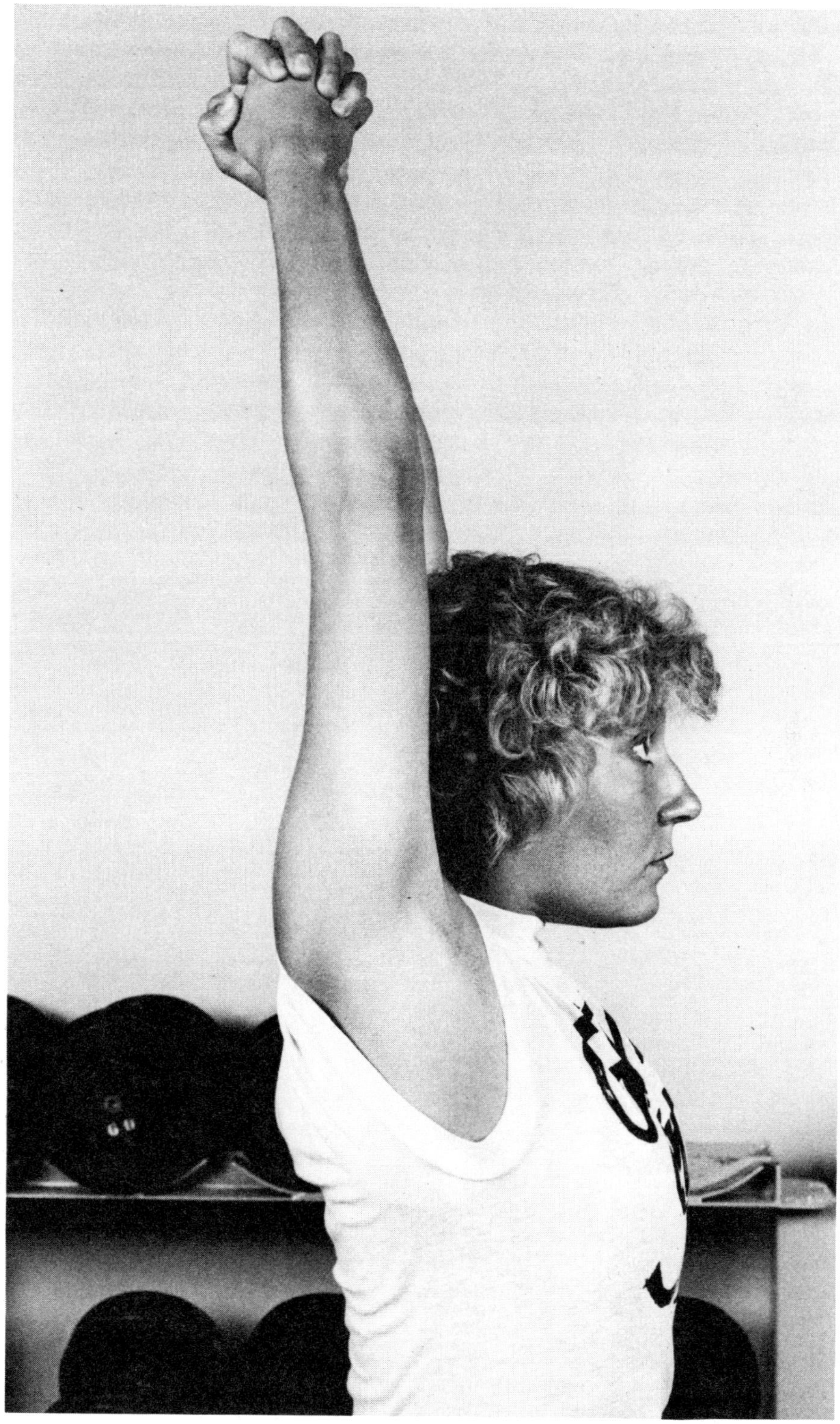

FOUR: SPECIFIC TRAINING GOALS

Why have training goals? Why should you take the time to write down the level of development or muscularity you want your chest to have? Because without a specific set of goals you're less likely to develop in the way you would like. A clearly defined plan will tell you which direction to take your training, and the training requirements necessary to realize your dreams.

Specific training goals will bring together your various desires, daydreams and images into a very real description of your ideal chest. The clearer the image, the greater chance you have of recognizing the result when you create it! If you are not absolutely sure of what you want, how are you going to recognize it when you achieve it?

Specific goals keep you motivated. It's easy for training intensity to lag and even go down without noticing. One day you notice you haven't seen many gains lately and then you realize "lately" has been a year or more. Long- and short-term goals will keep you on your toes (great for the calves, by the way) and never let you forget where you are going, even during the setbacks. Having deadlines is a great method, even if you don't quite make them, of keeping track of your progress.

It is much easier to cultivate the positive attitude necessary to create awesome muscular gains when you have goals. If you have 600,000 thoughts a day as the researchers

Called the Lion of Lebanon, 1983 Mr. Olympia Samir Bannout shows no flaws in this side chest pose.

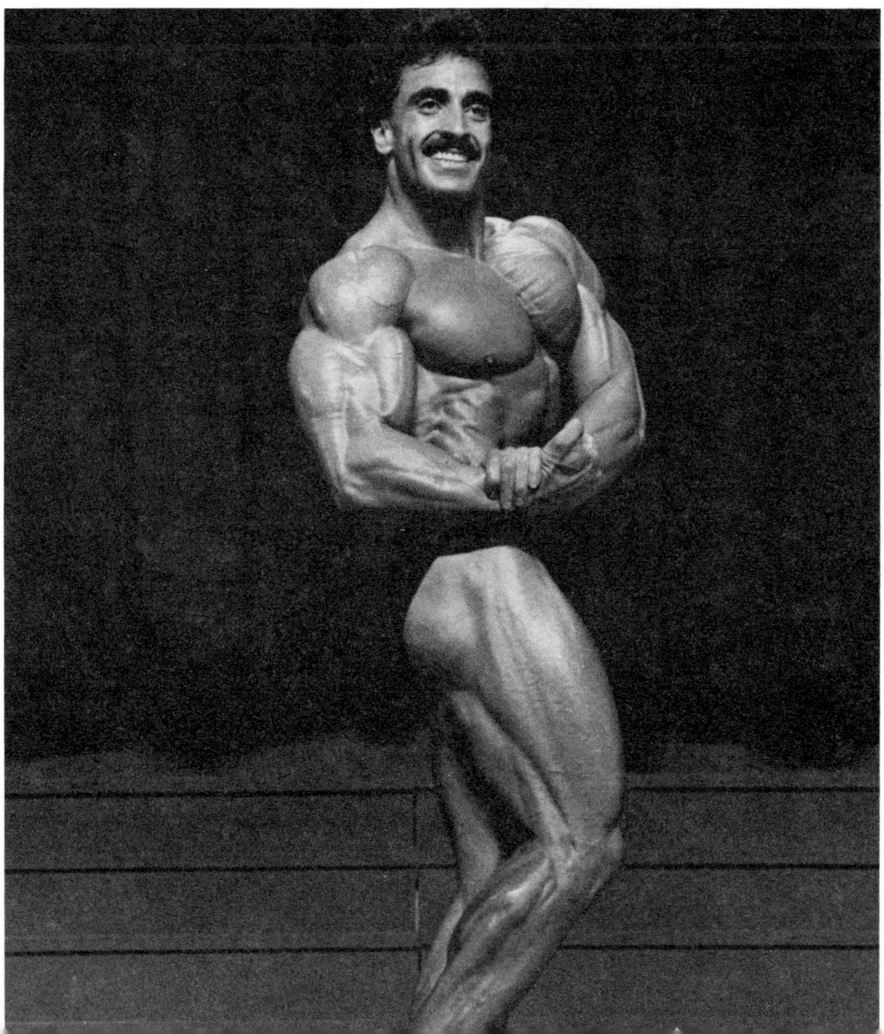

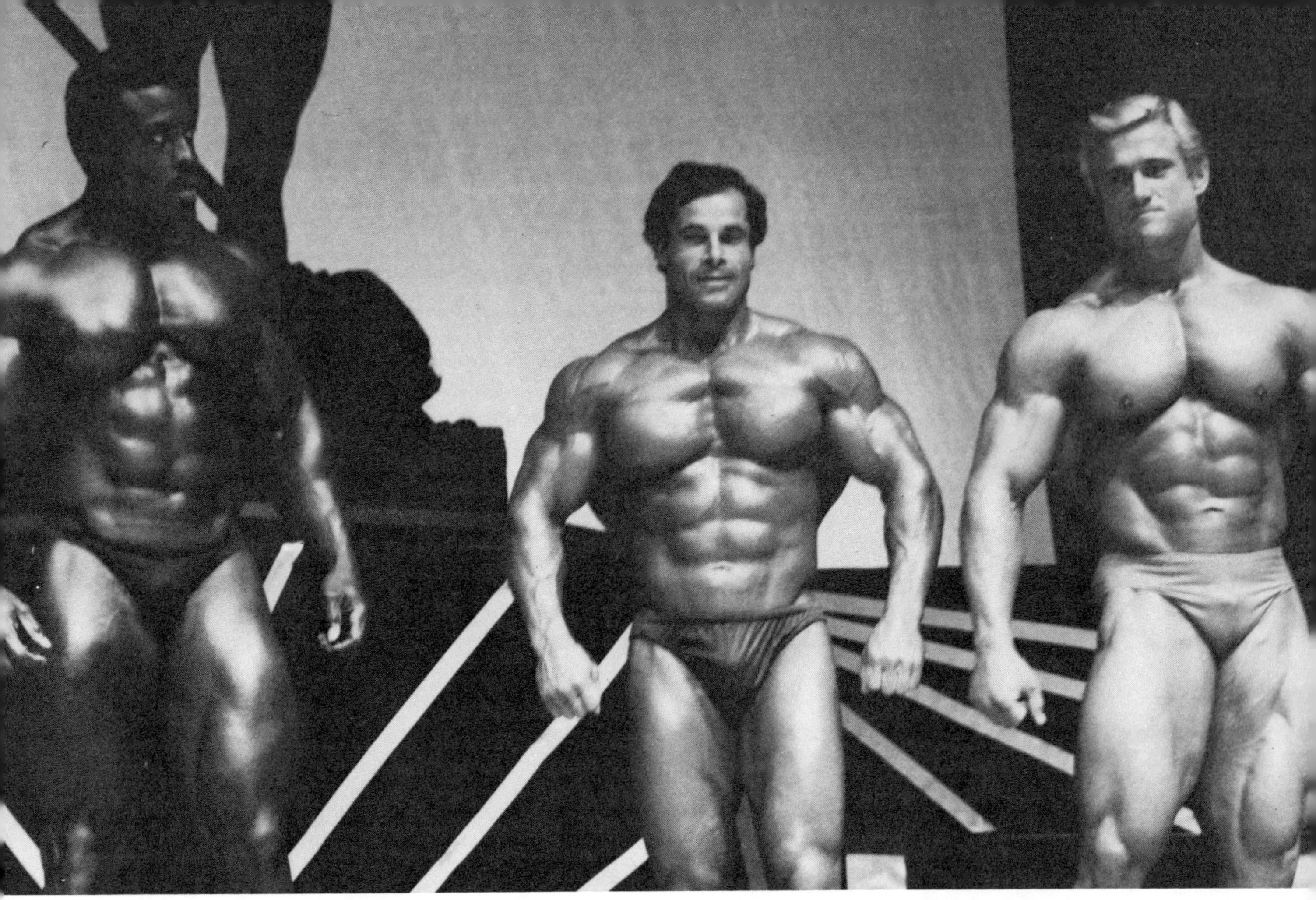

Three of the biggest names in the business: Roy Callander (left), Franco Columbu and Tom Platz show off the spectacular muscularity that has won each of them a place in bodybuilding history.

claim, and only 10 percent are negative thoughts, think how much time you spend programming yourself to fail! Most people have a much higher percentage of negative thoughts than 10 percent. It's not that hard to do. Observe how many times in a day you catch yourself thinking "I can't do this," or "I'll never have that." The thoughts and images we think to ourselves are called affirmations.

By focusing on specific goals, you keep positive affirmations ("I now have all the muscle mass I desire," is a great one) in the forefront and generate positive energy. Gains come much more easily when you believe in yourself 100 percent. Continually setting small goals and achieving them sets up a cycle of success and achievement that feeds upon itself. The more successful you are at a task, the more positive feedback you will receive, making the work to come that much easier. Winning ways produce winning ways! It's also easier to affirm success when you are experiencing it.

But goals need to be re-evaluated and altered as you achieve them. If your initial goal is to build the lower pecs, once achieved, you should change the goal or modify it. Train the lower pecs for density and muscularity once you have the size you desire.

Remember to have goals for both the long- and short-term. Let your long-term goal be extravagant, but keep your short-term goals as practical as possible. Don't be amazed when you find you can do more than you imagined.

Size, Density and Thickness Increases

Once you have the chest size you want, training for muscularity and muscle density will be the next step, and a rewarding one. Muscle mass is only part of the whole and must be treated as such. The muscle group must be thick, separated and dense to be complete. This is accomplished by high-intensity reps and total control of contractions. You must "get inside" the muscle and contract to the maximum throughout the entire range of motion. Slow negative reps, isolation training and Nautilus training accomplish this best.

Balancing the Upper and Lower Pecs

A problem of symmetry that plagues even the most advanced bodybuilders is lower pecs that overshadow the upper pecs. Excessive use of the bench press can cause or exacerbate this problem. Frank Zane believes excessively large lower pecs make the bodybuilder look effeminate. Of course, women bodybuilders that want to have more breast size and chest depth should do lower pec and bench press work. Incline work for a variety of rep schemes with dumbbell, barbell (narrow and wide grip) and pec dec work can correct an upper pec imbalance.

Definition and Muscularity

When working for definition and muscularity, the following is emphasized: continuous-tension exercises (especially cable and machine work), quality training (little or no rest between sets), peak contraction, posing practice (a little-known benefit to muscularity) and isolation training. Definition is most easily achieved when you have sufficient muscle mass. Training for definition before gaining enough pectoral mass is a waste of time. Striated, muscular pecs, however, are a sight to behold and are well worth the time necessary to create them.

Width Training

By emphasizing the outer edges of the pecs (and other muscles as well), you can bring an observer's eye out to the perimeter of the physique and enhance the appearance of width. A wide, flaring torso increases the size, depth and visual complexity of the physique and is a realistic goal everyone should include in his training. The best exercises for increasing the lower and outer edges of the chest are Flat Bench Flyes, wide (32-inch) Parallel Bar Dips with elbows out to the sides, Bench Presses with a wide grip, Decline Flyes and presses that stimulate the outer fibers of the sternal pecs. For someone with adequate outer, lower pecs, the same techniques can be applied with an incline bench to work on bringing out the upper, outer edge.

This chest pose of bodybuilder Lisa Elliot displays a dense muscularity that few women in the sport possess. The strong definition in the cleavage is the result of intense cross-pulley work.

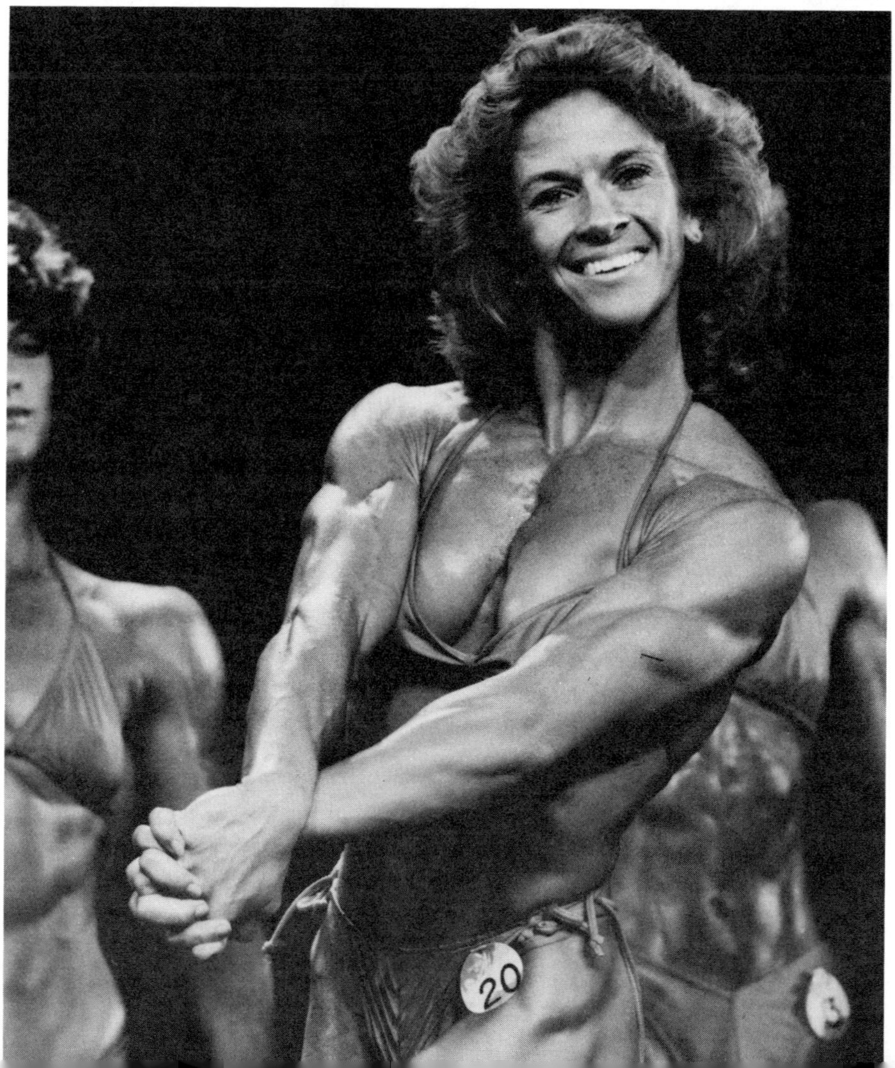

Strength Training and Power Training the Chest

This type of training is very satisfying because the results are so clear-cut—you can make the lift or you can't. Many people find this type of training more suitable than the isolation training and severe dieting necessary to compete in physique contests.

Challenging yourself with tests that require the same style of training you do in the gym can be much more satisfying when compared to the physique contestant who must compete with skills that are not the mainstay of training and are rarely practiced. The challenge most bodybuilders face daily is trial by iron. The skill and art of bodybuilding requires a mastery of movements and strength that will never be demonstrated in a bodybuilding contest.

Posing is a valid art form, but it's not what got the bodybuilder into his sport. Strength training is thought by many to be the purest form of weightlifting; you're training for yourself and your own goals. The rewards are constant, unlike bodybuilding where you might compete only once a year.

Powerlifting and Olympic lifting are gaining popularity. Women have begun to enter the sport en masse now that it's an acceptable form of training for them. The results are amazing. Bev Francis of Australia, weighing 181 pounds, has bench pressed 330 pounds!

Powerlifting (Squat, Bench Press and Deadlift done for one repetition using maximum weight) in-

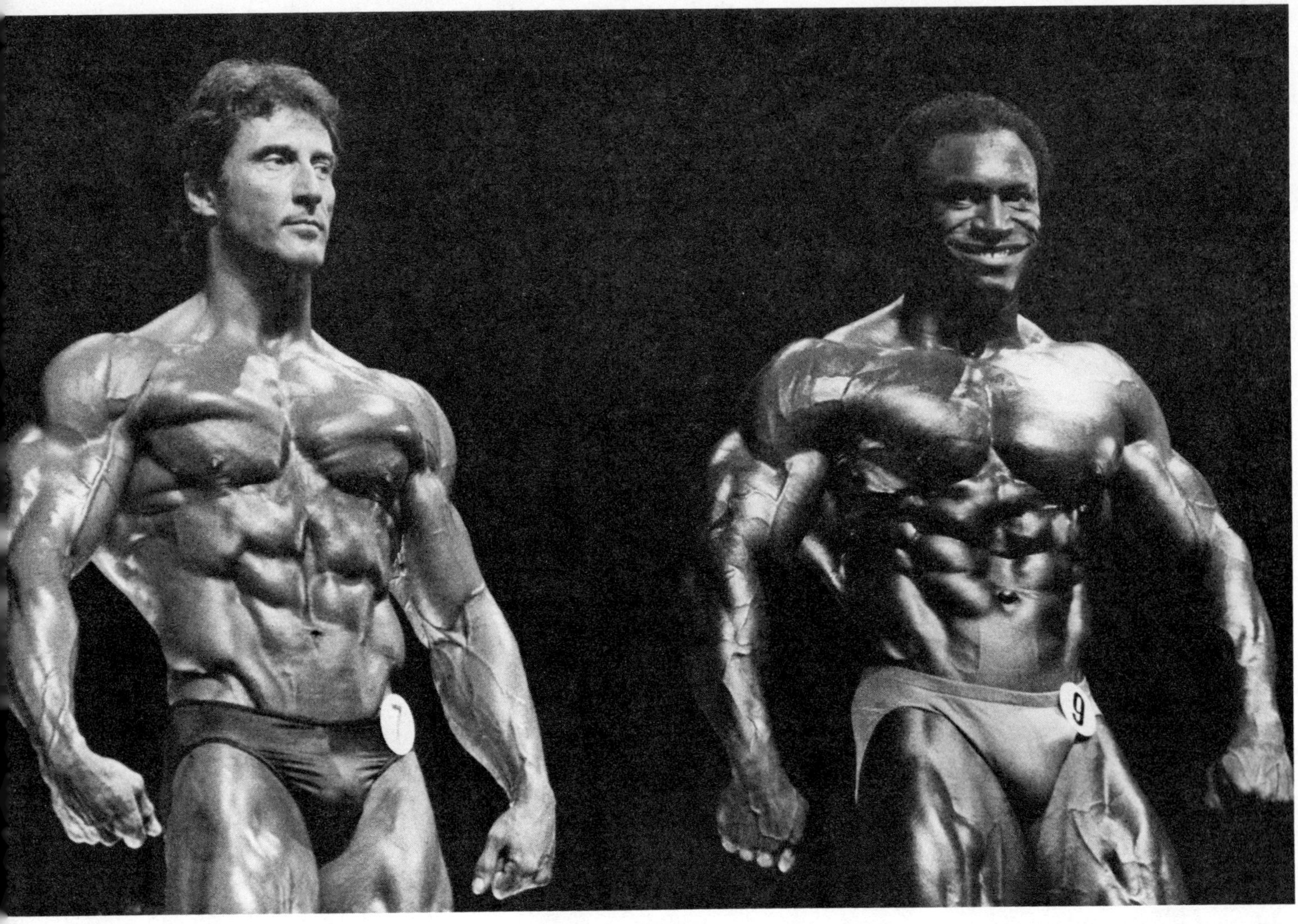

Bodybuilding superstars Frank Zane and Lee Haney seem to be suggesting that it's what's up front that counts.

volves no momentum and properly should be called Strengthlifting, because of the heavy weights and slow lifting speeds. Olympic lifting (Snatch, Clean and Jerk) involves speed and power.

Very basic exercises, heavy loads (85 to 95 percent of one rep max) for low reps are the key to gaining total body strength and power.

Lower Pec Development and Fat Reduction

Many men have fat deposits in the lower pec area. More than a few of my students have had this problem. Usually the way fat is deposited determines where fat is lost first when you begin training. "Last on first off" is the rule of thumb; many men developed fat on their lower pecs when they were adolescents, making it fairly difficult to remove and often necessitating a reduction of body fat to get rid of it.

My training partner has had excellent results developing his lower pecs and reducing body fat in the low pec area using a training routine that works all areas of the pecs during his chest and triceps training. He does a wide variety of rep schemes, exercises and angle training and uses a low-fat, low-calorie diet. He has increased muscle mass by emphasizing his lower pecs. Decline bench work blasts this area well. His fat loss has been accomplished through an increase in muscle mass, a subsequent increase in metabolism, and aerobic training.

▶

Lee Haney, still in his 20s, is one of the youngest of the professional male bodybuilders. His remarkable combination of symmetry, proportion and unbelievable mass will certainly win him many more of the top titles.

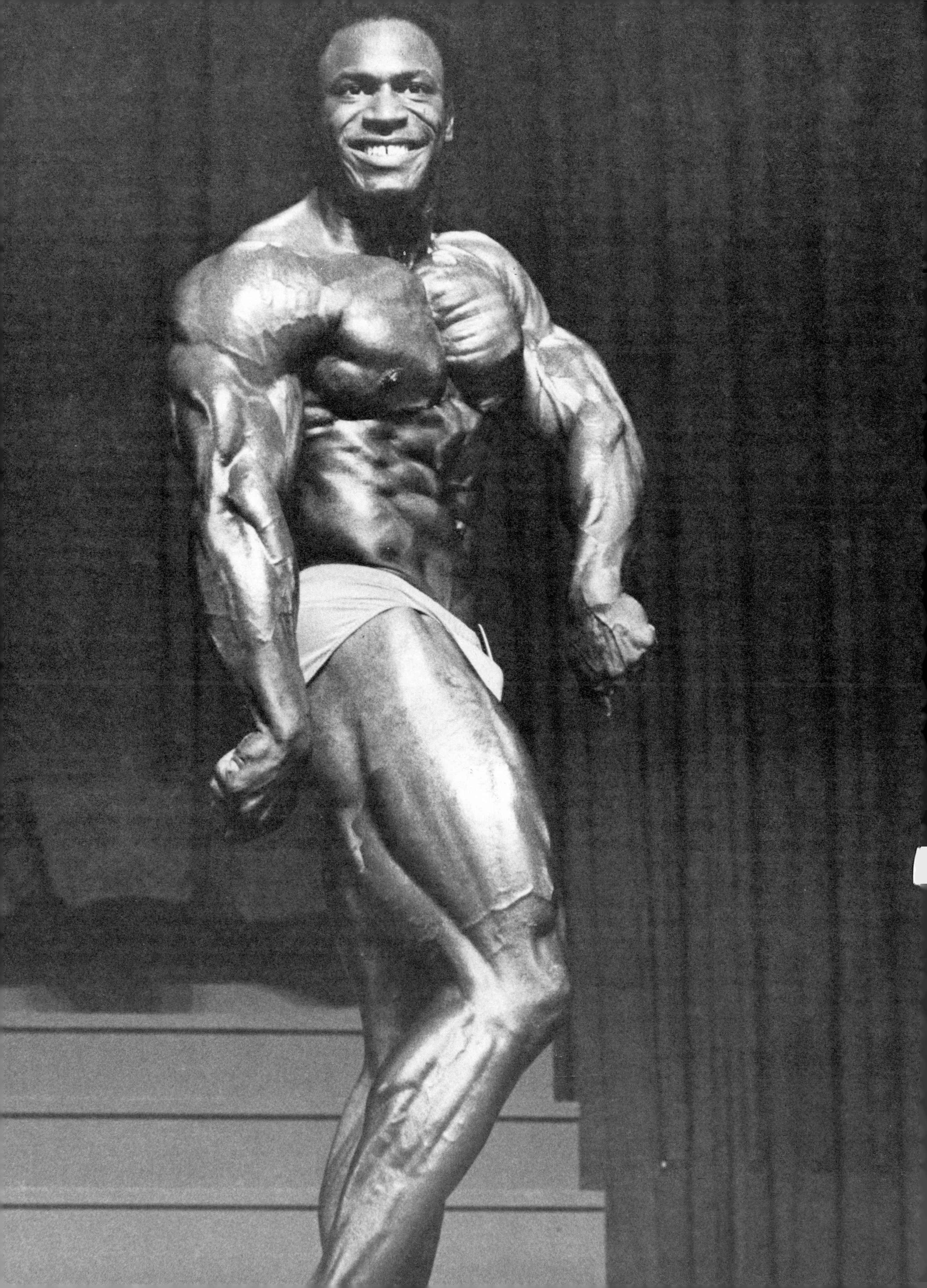

FIVE: EQUIPMENT AND APPARATUS

The more diverse the movements, the more muscle fibers will be exposed, and their development will be more complete. You don't need a complete line of machines to make progress in your training, but a variety of angled benches and cable systems will make training more exciting and creative.

The various types of pec decs or chest machines are almost indispensable for thick inner pec development. It's the most comfortable way to work this area. Dual cable crossover systems make carving deep lines on the chest almost fun, with their smooth pulleys and strong peak contractions.

Mainly you need the diversity of machines and benches as you get into more advanced training levels. Beginners make excellent progress because their muscles have never been exposed to high-intensity contractions. Basic, straight line barbell and dumbbell training provides more than enough stress to beginners' muscles as they try to adjust to the shifting workload.

Because the motions are uncoordinated when you're learning, each rep goes up slightly differently, so there is a wide range of muscle adaptation. As you become more coordinated with your lifting, the muscles need more diverse lines of pull and angle training for stimulation. This can be accomplished by adding exercises or using the same machine in a different fashion.

Dr. Tom McLaughlin of the National Strength Research Center at Auburn University believes that changing the style of an exercise keeps the adaptation process working. McLaughlin's studies indicate that changing the stance, grip, tempo of reps or the angle of the exercise, even slightly, can shock the muscles into new growth. The muscle adapts to stress very quickly by becoming more efficient. The more efficient the movement, the less stress is transferred to the muscles and the less stimulation that occurs. McLaughlin also believes that there is no one exercise program that you can stay on forever. He says, "No fixed workout, no matter how perfect, will work for very long. Any training program that does not effectively and systematically utilize change will eventually lead to overtraining."

I agree with the doctor. By changing the style of the exercises or the exercise itself each workout, I have found that my body is kept in a constant state of growth. Keeping the body constantly forced to adapt to new motions by using unfamiliar angles and grooves continually stimulates the body into more complete compensations.

This system of constant change works well for me. I can stay with exercises that I know best, and I can work the weak areas of the muscle much longer. Once I have found an exercise that I can feel in a certain part of the muscle and it brings results, I am reluctant not to use it. Changing the machine, angle or grip allows me to constantly use an exercise without growing stale.

I also train each body part only once a week, which allows me even more leeway in reusing exercises. Provided enough time has lapsed, 10 to 14 days, the muscle loses enough efficiency to gain from repeated exercises. As McLaughlin says, though, there is no one perfect routine and the only thing constant is change.

I still like to master a variety of difficult free weight movements, the art form of bodybuilding. The skill level involved in squatting or deadlifting with heavy weight for high reps intrigues and challenges me. I want to be able to do something with an incredibly developed body.

Most bodybuilders will do best by changing some of the exercises in the routine every four to six weeks, and changing the grip, stance or tempo of the basic exercise more often (one to two weeks). The more advanced you get, the more esoteric you can become. Supinating One-Arm Peak Contraction Cable Crossovers might help Mr. Olympia put the finishing touches on his pecs, but bench presses will do the beginner a lot more good.

The theory of needing constantly changing angles and stress for growth is one reason why free weight training is considered superior to machine training. Machines usually lock you into a set pathway. Once your central nervous system has adapted to that particular movement, increasing the weight might not be enough to get the stimulation you need. Changing the type of machine will help, but, ultimately, free weight training brings the best results.

TRAINING FACILITIES

You can't get into a serious competitive-level bodybuilding program training on your patio with vinyl weights. If that's what you want to train with, you'll have to reconsider your goals.

Serious training programs require serious gyms. Commercial gyms, like Gold's and World's, are franchised and can be found in most large cities. Commerical gyms with Nautilus and other machine equipment are opening at a steady pace around the country.

But even if you don't have access to a modern gym with all the latest equipment, you can get excellent results from the basic set-up of an adjustable bench and an Olympic barbell set. You don't even need dumbbells. The wide variety of machines and benches at gyms make for more interesting workouts, but the movements necessary for muscle growth can be obtained with a basic set of weights. It is ultimately the mind and genetics that determine how big, shapely and muscular you get.

You can alter the form on the barbell bench press just by changing grip width and varying the spot where you lower the bar on your chest. A limitless number of variations is available with basic compound movements. For competition, however, more equipment would help your chances greatly.

If you are a powerlifter, it is easier to set up a complete home gym because less equipment is needed than for bodybuilding. But never train alone, especially when doing heavy bench presses or squats; you can misjudge your strength and get pinned by the bar. Deaths have occurred from misjudging how much weight can be lifted while bench pressing and dropping the bar on the neck.

RECOVERY TIME

Recovery time increases geometrically with training intensity. The harder you train, the more rest you need. Training two hours a day is not just twice as difficult as training one hour a day, but at least four times as hard! Your strength can increase, from your first day in the gym to peak performance, as much as 300 percent. Your recovery ability, however, will increase only about 50 percent.

As we've discussed, a stronger muscle takes more out of the system when trained intensely. For example, a 20-inch arm going to muscular failure on a set of heavy curls takes significantly more time to recover compared to a 12-inch arm. This must be taken into account when planning your training program. Do not allow yourself to train more than you can recover from.

In your beginning training, you are not strong enough to deplete your ability to recover fully, so you can train muscles three times per week.

You cannot train large body parts with high intensity and expect to jump from the gym to work without transition and recovery time, so even more time is required as you advance. Most athletes will benefit from a hard depletion workout followed by a day of rest. Alternating heavy and light days allows you to recuperate.

PEER SUPPORT

Before you begin a training program, be sure you have the support of your friends or the important person in your life. You will eliminate a lot of problems from the start by stating your intentions—how much you will train in the gym, how much training will take from your personal life. Just because you have dedicated your life to growing incredible pecs doesn't mean anyone else is going to understand or care. This is especially true if your friend doesn't train.

The demands of bodybuilding and strength training can try the patience of the most loving and supporting individuals. The more understanding and support you get, the easier your task will be.

SIX: AVOIDING INJURY

To increase your flexibility as fast as possible, contract the muscles while you're stretching. When the contraction is voluntary, sent by the person stretching and resisted by a training partner, it's called PNF stretching or proprioceptor neuromuscular facilitation.

PNF stretching involves stretching to the point of pain, contracting the muscle to fool nerve receptors and then relaxing, with your training partner helping you further into the stretch. The contractions should last six seconds and you can do as many reps as you can stand.

SHOULDER STRETCHES

Because most injuries to the pecs also directly or indirectly involve the deltoids, it is vital that you increase the flexibility of this important joint. This is very easy, because the shoulder joint is a relatively shallow ball-and-socket joint. The construction that makes it so unstable and prone to injury (wide range of motion, lack of structural stabilizers) also makes it very easy to stretch. The key stretching tools are a towel and a training partner.

For stretching the shoulders by yourself, the best method is overhead stretches with a towel. This stretch is very popular with gymnasts, who use sticks instead of towels. Towels are more pliable and easier to use. First, loosen the shoulders by doing arm circles forward and backward, starting with very small circles, progressing to larger ones and then returning to the smallest circles you can make. Do all the forward circles before the backward circles. Circle the arms until the shoulders feel loose and warm.

Take a regular-size bath towel and roll it into a cigar shape. Grasp both ends of the towel with your hands in an overgrip (palms facing your body) and lift both arms as high as possible without leaning back. This can be done sitting or standing. When you reach the

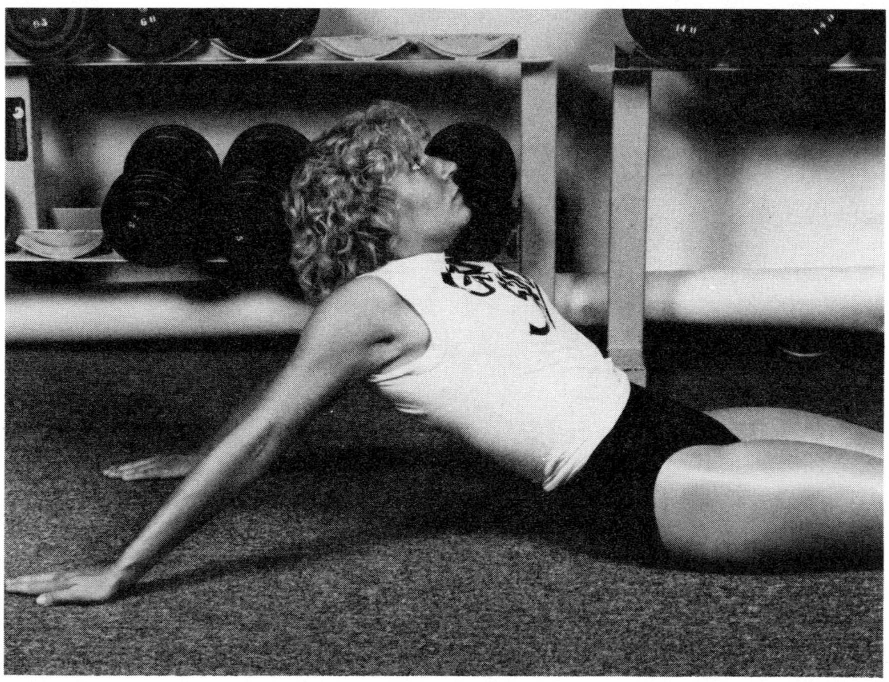

This movement stretches the front portion of the shoulder girdle. Sit with your arms locked at your sides and your legs extended in front of you, then slide your hips forward.

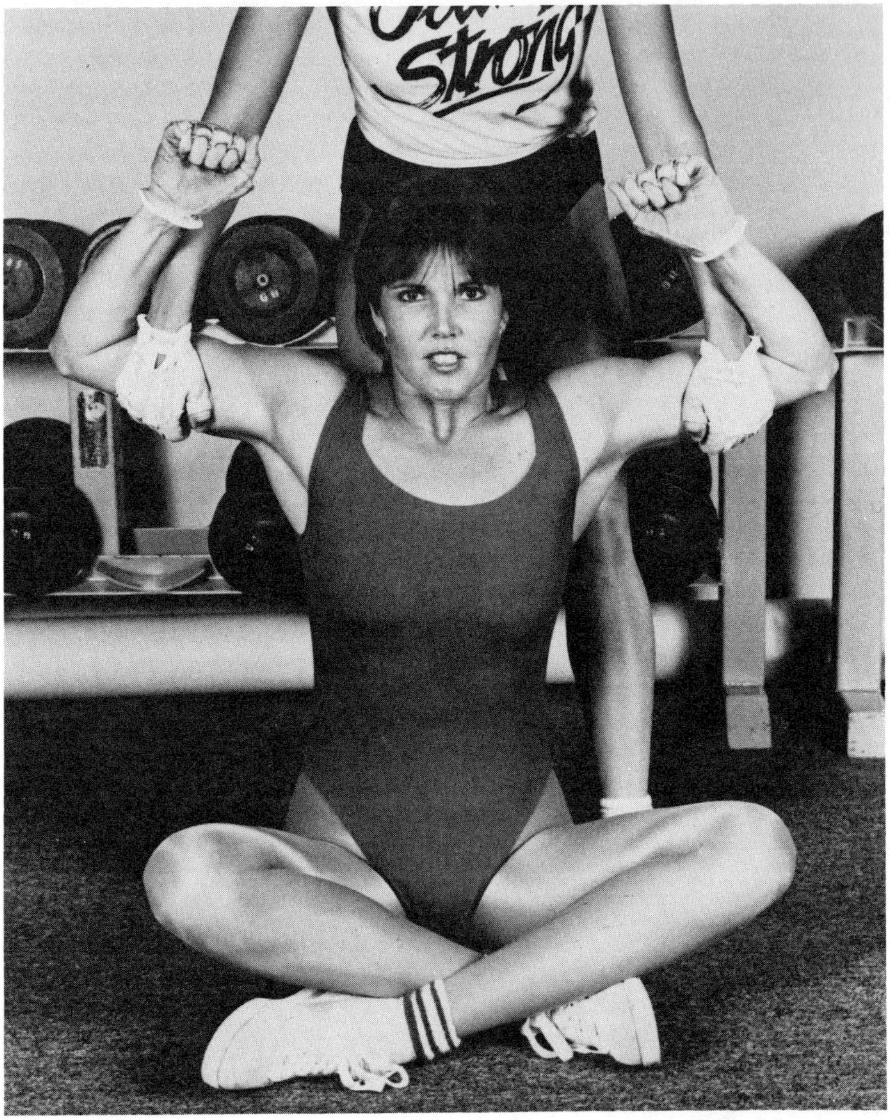

A training partner can help you get a good shoulder stretch. For this exercise your training partner pulls your shoulders up and back.

point where you can't lift the towel any higher and still can hold the position, hold it for 20 seconds and work up to one minute. Repeat three times.

To work the shoulders from the other direction, sit on the floor with your hands behind you, fingers pointing behind you, hands shoulder-width apart. Slowly slide your body away from the arms until you reach a point of maximum stretch that can be held. Be careful not to lock the arms, as this exercise can be hard on the elbows. Hold for 20 seconds and repeat three times.

It is much easier to stretch the shoulders with a partner. While you are in an upright sitting position on the floor, arms overhead, have your partner reach through and around your arms. Have him brace your back with his knee. You should pull down as if you were doing a straight-arm pulldown on the lat machine. Have your partner resist for six seconds and utilize the PNF technique for three to four contractions. After each contraction/relaxation, have your partner pull your shoulders behind your head, keeping them as close as possible. You must be very very gentle with all shoulder stretches! Never force any position.

To isolate the pecs with PNF, have your partner hold your arms from the back again, at the elbows. Place your arms in the same position as for Vertical Flyes. Contract the pecs against your partner's resistance. Hold for six seconds, release, stretch further and repeat.

This is a very simple, fast and productive method of increasing your chest and shoulder flexibility, as well as warming up the shoulder/pec area.

TORSO WARMUP EXERCISES

It is vital to get blood into the torso with low-intensity stretching and contractions before exercising the muscles with heavy weights and high-intensity contractions. The muscles and joints must be prepared for the heavy work. Walking into the gym and doing three quick sets of Bench Presses before hitting max weights is not the best way to increase strength or size.

An excellent warmup for the upper torso muscles (besides general aerobics for the whole system) is low-intensity sets of light exercises such as Push-ups, Pulldowns, light Bench Presses and Dips, focusing entirely on getting blood into the area and doing some light contractions. The exercises should be done with about 40 percent of your usual 10-rep max weight.

I like to use Pulldowns on a lat machine as a chest-day warmup. They work the antagonist muscles of the back and in so doing really stretch the chest. I use high reps, about eight to the front, then eight behind the neck, and eight half-reps where I just pull down from the shoulder blades; I leave my biceps out of the action. One or two sets of these, along with the PNF or static towel stretches, and I'm ready for some chest work.

MOMENTUM: WHY YOU SHOULDN'T "CHEAT"

The most destructive training technique is the use of excessive "cheating," also known as momentum. By throwing weights around using body English and speed to overcome fatigue, weakness or poor leverage, you get very good at throwing weights around, but that's all. Meanwhile, you increase stress to the joints and the chance of injury. Even with very light weights, the load on the tendons and joints can be increased astronomically by using momentum.

The cheating principles of advanced bodybuilding are for very advanced bodybuilders. Power training is essential but only with perfect form. You never see good powerlifters using sloppy technique and loose form. Their benches must be done with a strict pause on the chest—no bouncing for them!

Forced reps done with strict form and enough assistance to finish off the movement are safe for increasing intensity. Never bounce weights off your chest; if no spotters are available, use lighter weights or machines.

Learning to use only the contractile force of the isolated muscles to raise and lower weight is the best way to increase muscle mass and decrease the chance of injury. As soon as momentum is used, the chances of injury increase.

PYRAMID REP SCHEME: THE SAFETY FACTOR

There are many different theories how to train the chest and how to get to your heaviest set of the workout. Some trainers and athletes advocate doing warmup sets with very light weights until the area is "glowing with warmth," and then going right to their heaviest weight for the exercise. After this set, each proceeding set gets lighter to work the muscle with the heaviest weights when the energy reserves are highest. I have tried this method and it works, but the major drawback is the risk of injury. If you are lucky you can go for a relatively long time using this method without getting hurt. But as you get stronger and the weights on that first set get heavier, the ratio shifts; I've found that I get injured much easier this way.

It takes a number of progressively heavier sets to work up to my heaviest weight safely. When I start too heavy, my form is never as good as when I work up slower; neither is my coordination or strength. Doing three fairly heavy sets before going for a very heavy six-rep set, and then another, should tire me out, but that doesn't happen.

The first three sets are done to the maximum, each with the heaviest weights possible for the required reps. But by the time I get to the last two sets, my strength is consistently better than if I take token weight jumps to my max weight. On the first exercise of the day I also take two extra-light warmups. It works like this:

Set 1—warmup, 1 × 20 very light

Set 2—warmup, 1 × 10 fairly close to my starting weight

Set 3—first real set, 1 × 15

Set 4—set two (real), 1 × 12, then 1 × 10, 1 × 18, 1 × 6.

REDUCING THE RISK OF INJURY

Full Range of Motion

Some people shy away from full ranges of motion because they think the stretch is dangerous. This is only true if you are inflexible through a particular range of motion. Take each rep as far as possible into the stretch, because this is what is primarily responsible for muscle gains. Heavy overload is required throughout the largest range of motion possible. What do you do if your range of motion is limited? Increase it by arduous flexibility training. As your joint flexibility increases, so does your strength, muscle shape and size.

Using the Body as a Base

One of the easiest ways to injure yourself when training the chest is to struggle under weights that are too heavy. I see it every day in the gym. Someone is always doing his reps with atrocious form, writhing under the weight as if he were a fish on a hook. He moves his feet just when he needs to be driving through the legs; he twists his head and neck from side to side or tries to gain leverage by bridging under the bar on his neck! With "style" like that, it's only a question of time when you are going to be injured.

When going for the heaviest possible weights in any power exercise, especially in power benching, tightening and locking the body into the power position is essential for safe and powerful benching. This is one reason why strong bench pressers are so massive and powerful-looking. Using the heaviest weights they can, the entire body comes into play for each lift. No muscle gets to slide.

Such form contributes to a big bench but, more importantly, it protects the lifter from injury. If you can't use a weight under control and with good form, find a lighter weight. Remember, the idea is development, both of size and strength. The only way to improve is by controlling your weights, not having them control you. Your strength will fluctuate almost daily, but maintaining form will always guarantee that you are getting as much out of the motion as possible.

Weight Selection and Natural Biorhythms

"Some days," Grand Prix Winner Scott Wilson says, "a bodybuilder can motivate himself to squat with 500 pounds for 10 reps. Then there are other times when he can't motivate himself to do one! What's that

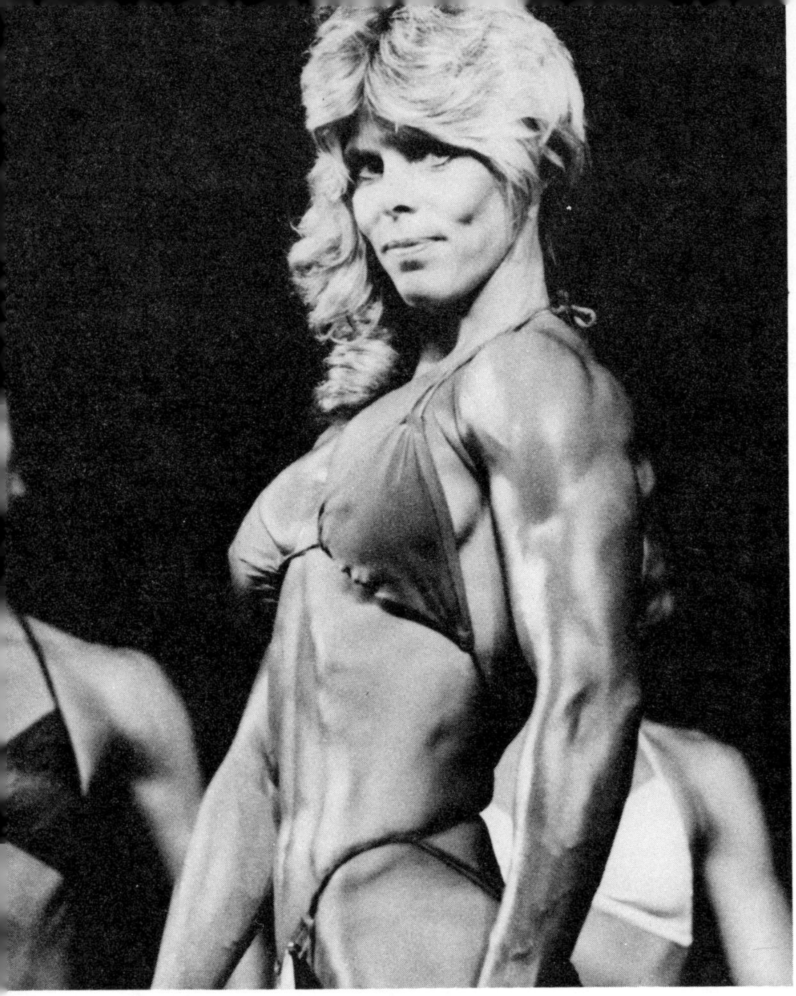

Leslie Kozlow is one of the most sensual posers in women's bodybuilding. Her combination of strength, muscularity and femininity continues to win her top titles in women's physique.

about? It's the mind. The mind gives out before the body; it's the mind you have to train the hardest. That's what will take you to bodybuilding success."

The point, Scott believes, is that although the body's strength fluctuates because of emotional and physical variables, training with this knowledge enables you to go to your limit and stimulate muscle growth. All you do is accept where you are in a workout and go with the flow, taking it to the limit for the day.

"All that really counts," Scott believes, "is that last rep. Your body doesn't know whether there's 200 pounds or 400 pounds on the bar; it only knows whether it can do it or not. All last reps are hard."

Problems can arise if you try to speed up progress by circumventing this law of nature. Remember, keeping flexible with exercises and proper weight selections can maintain progress much longer than shooting for the fast gains. Designing a regimented schedule that you keep to no matter what, is like asking injury over for dinner with an engraved invitation and sending a limousine to pick it up.

Your body works in cycles and the more you learn about how your personal cycle fluctuates, the easier it will be on your head (ego) and the faster and longer you will progress. The key is to go as heavy as possible but recognize that when your strength levels are down you are much more injury-prone. Train as hard as you can, but don't get hurt using weight you usually handle when feeling terrific.

If the schedule calls for a 10-pound jump in the bench but you know that 20 will go, go for it. But in the same vein, if it calls for 10 pounds and you did the last set with a lot of help, choose a more appropriate weight. You can't grow muscle if you are injured and can't train. Listen to your body and you'll be training for a long time.

Some factors that affect your strength and energy level are controllable. Most of them involve changes in the daily routine. Drastic differences in workout time or patterns can alter your strength by 50 percent or more. I recently had to train at 7 p.m. instead of my usual 9 a.m. because of my training partner's job change. I couldn't believe how bad the change was for me. My strength and energy, after working and waiting all day, was gone!

I spent a good deal of the day "saving" energy and adrenaline for the evening workout. I had to train on a full colon, which makes a world of difference if you are not used to it. The entire day I was anxiously waiting for the training session. But by the time I got in the gym, the last thing I wanted to do was train! I was used to relaxing at this time and reading.

Here are some of the common variables that can cause an increased risk of injury and decreased strength in your training:

1) changing the time of the workout drastically.

2) changing the order of exercises. This seems academic but you'd be surprised. People who change the order and do their benches in the middle of the chest workout instead of the beginning are amazed to find they can't lift anything near what they could when they are fresh.

3) changing the diet before training. Eating a heavy meal or foods you're unaccustomed to before training can have disastrous effects. Try to stay with foods you know work for you.

4) increasing or decreasing your sleep. Getting less sleep than normal is one of the major strength reducers. Usually it is not the immediate day after you miss sleep that your strength suffers but 48 hours later. Getting too much sleep, such as taking an unscheduled nap, can make you groggy and lethargic.

5) recreational drugs. Someone comes in on Monday after a "vigorous" weekend partying and finds that his strength is so low he needs to hide. In the gym you can run but you can't hide, and if you play too hard you won't be very strong for quite a while.

You can keep yourself injury-free (or as close to it as humanly possible) by:

1) raising the body's temperature before stretching or lifting weights.

2) doing enough flexibility training to achieve optimal levels of joint and muscle flexibility.

3) doing low-intensity general exercises before the heavy work.

4) using an inverted pyramid rep scheme to get to the very heavy weight slowly and safely.

5) controlling and resisting the negative portions of reps.

6) never using momentum to lift the weight.

7) using a full range of motion.

8) using the body as a strength base (no wiggling!).

9) choosing weights that are in accordance with your strength levels each workout.

10) adjusting weights and workout load for external variables that you cannot control (change of training time, sleep, and so on).

11) listening to the natural rhythm and strength fluctuations of the body and modifying the routine around them.

12) keeping changes in your training routine to a minimum.

SEVEN: BASIC ROUTINES

The basic routines that you begin your chest training with are extremely important as they provide the base from which all your future muscle mass gains will originate. If your base is shaky, your future gains will not be as impressive or quick in coming as they could be.

Beginners, intermediate and advanced trainers all should have a core routine that they know covers the bases and works all the area of the pecs without causing overtraining. Quality can never be supplanted by quantity in bodybuilding. If you can't do one set properly with contraction control and concentration, 20 sloppy sets won't make things any better.

The time it takes to master the basic exercises and the variations for intermediate and advanced training will pay dividends until the final rep of your bodybuilding career. These basic exercises are done by all the champs all the time, even in the precontest cycle; that's how important they are!

If you are new to weight training, the first thing you must learn is the basic movements and how they are done. The first weeks or months, focus almost entirely on form, with weight a secondary consideration. In the beginning of your training, the first strength increases will almost entirely be because of learning. Performing each exercise efficiently, with no extraneous motions, and focusing on the muscle contracting is the goal of beginning chest training.

The basic exercises revolve around pressing movements with dumbbells and barbells. I prefer dumbbell work for beginners for a number of reasons: There is no chance of being pinned under a heavy bar; dumbbells are unwieldy, requiring you to control not only the vertical pressing motion, but also all forward, backward and sideways motions; you can use fairly light weight and still get a great workout.

Pressing involves not only the pecs but the triceps, shoulders and to some degree the lats and neck. This makes presses the most economical exercise for the chest and upper body mass and strength in general. Isolation exercises are not needed until the intermediate level where you are doing a split routine. Even then, basic compound presses should be at the front of your workout.

The best beginning exercise that stretches the muscles (length contraction) is the Pullover. The presses are also essential for creating the largest mass gains because they work the muscle hardest in the mid-range position, stressing the large muscle belly the greatest and returning the greatest size increases of all the exercises.

Intermediate and advanced bodybuilders need to concern themselves with peak contraction, isolation and shaping movements. The beginner just has to get strong.

BEGINNING CHEST ROUTINE

	Sets	Reps
Flat Bench Dumbbell Bench Press	1-4	15
Dumbbell Pullover	1-4	15
Seated Dumbbell Shoulder Press	1-4	15
Parallel Bar Dip	1-4	max

Now you might notice that 1) there is an awful lot of work for a beginning program, 2) not all of these exercises are direct chest exercises, and 3) the reps are very high. All of this is intentional.

Each of the exercises works the chest from a different angle, but, because they are all compound exercises, they also work the surrounding muscles of the torso. This is the best way for beginners to work the chest without overtraining it.

The basic motion that must be learned is pressing. Overhead presses, such as Seated Dumbbell Presses, work the upper chest as well as the deltoids. The deltoids and triceps are intimately involved in any type of chest press, be it with a barbell, dumbbell or machine.

Pullovers work not only the upper chest but the lats, triceps, deltoids and rib cage. The Dips put stress on the lower pecs and triceps, all of which need to be strong in order to do advanced chest work.

The repetitions are high because it is essential that the beginner learn the basic form as quickly as possible. High reps accomplish this best. The high reps also increase circulation and start the capillary production necessary for proper nutrient flow to the muscles. And they strengthen the joints and connective tissue. High reps develop endurance and teach you to deal with the pain of waste product buildup (the burn). But this is not to say that you should avoid using progressive resistance. Add weight each set if you can, just keep the reps up to 15. When you can do all four sets of 15, increase your starting weight by 10 percent.

Flat Bench Dumbbell Bench Press

Lie flat on an exercise bench with the dumbbells at arm's length above you, plates touching as if the dumbbells formed a solid barbell. Palms are facing forward. Keep your shoulders pulled back flat on the bench. Keep the hips down and the feet flat on the ground. The chin should be tucked into the chest and the upper back slightly arched. The glutes are on the bench. Lower the dumbbells, keeping the hands over the elbows until you reach maximum stretch, at pec level or below. Push the dumbbells back to arm's length and resist the urge to change the position of the torso. Keep the upper back arched by pulling tight on the shoulder blades. Focus on contracting the pecs.

Dumbbell Pullover

This technique was discussed in Chapter 3. The key points to remember are to keep the hips down, the torso rotated upward and to relax the triceps so that maximum stretch can be achieved. Tilting the dumbbell slightly forward as it comes overhead will bring the upper pecs into play.

Pullovers can also be performed with a dumbbell as well as a bar. For this variation, place your thumbs around the handle and rest your palms against one of the inside plates. ▼

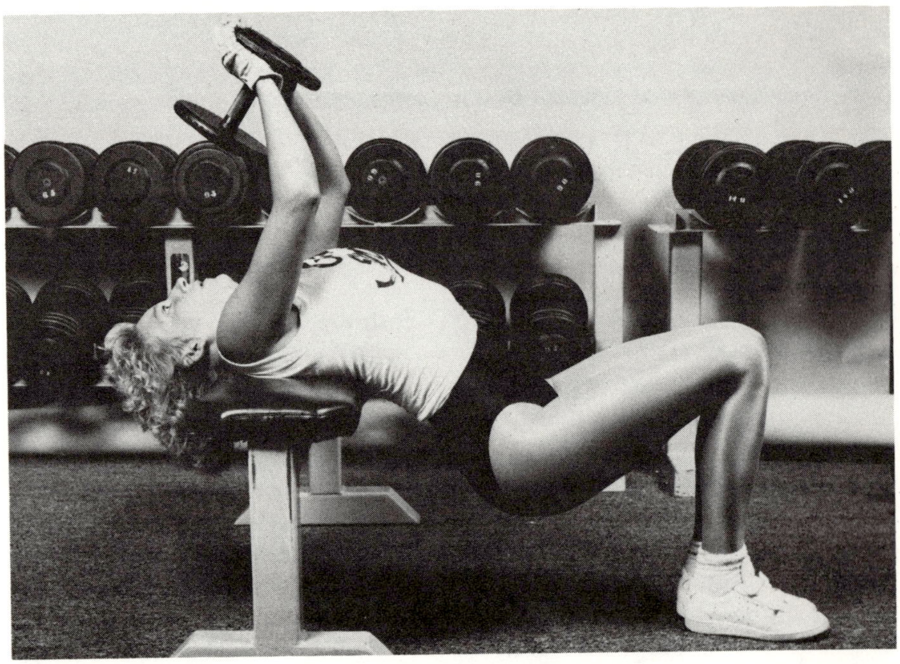

This is the stretched position of the Dumbbell Pullover. The elbows should be slightly bent at the completion of this movement. ▶

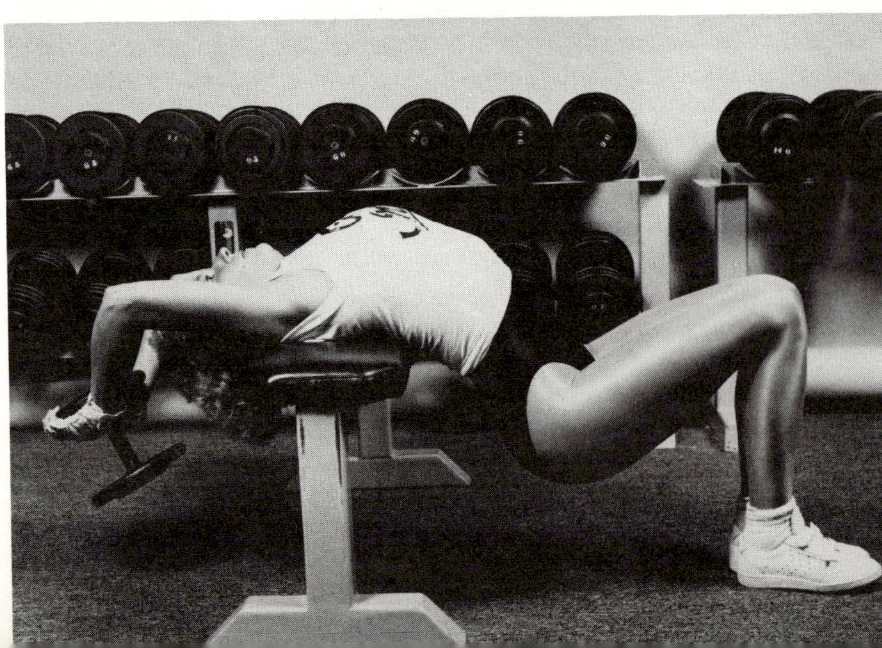

Chris Kiesman demonstrates the starting position of the Dumbbell Press. To maximize overall deltoid development, keep your elbows out to your sides rather than in front.

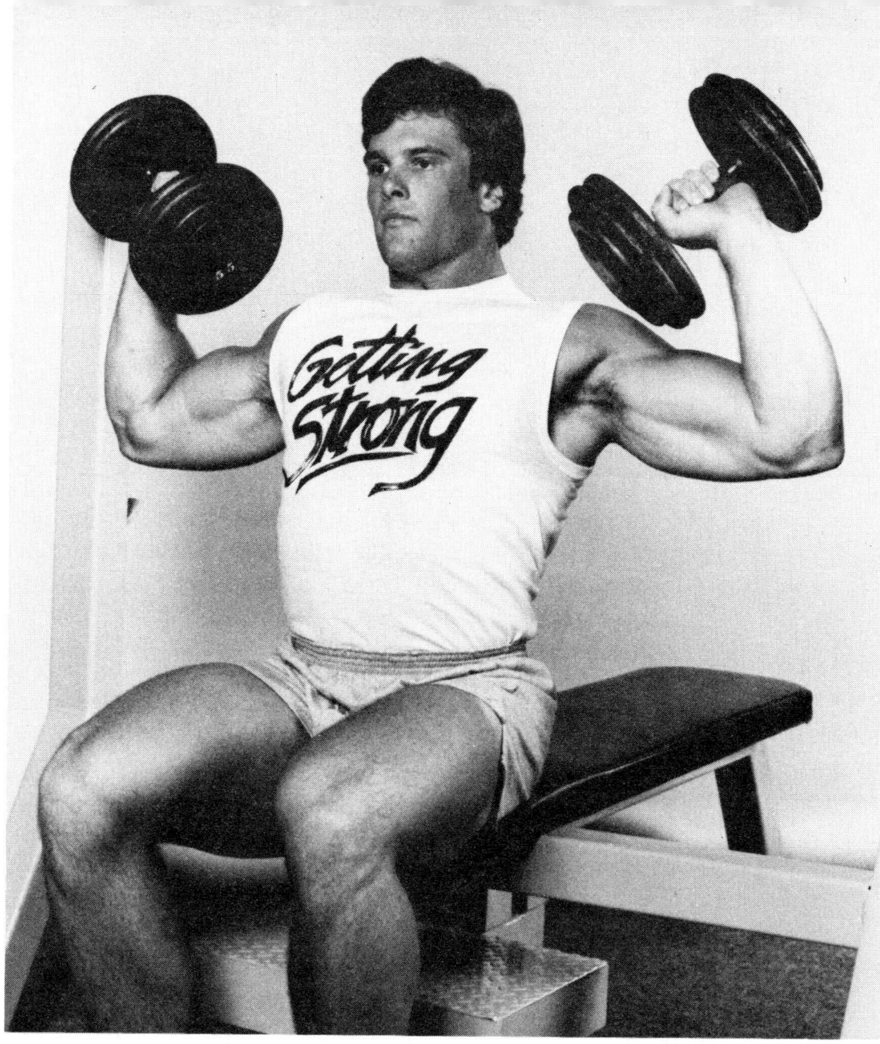

Seated Dumbbell Shoulder Press

Sit upright on an exercise bench, with the feet spread apart and firmly on the floor. Keep the back as straight as possible. You should feel as if you have a steel rod down your spine. Start with the dumbbells at shoulder level. Press them overhead. Keep the dumbbells back as far as possible, as if they were a solid bar and you were pressing it behind your neck.

Parallel Bar Dip

Start on the parallel bars, arms straight, hips bent forward slightly, knees bent. Lower slowly into the full dip position, leaning slightly forward as you descend. The elbows go out to the side. Keep the chin on the chest and the back slightly round. Push back up to the start position, and contract the pecs hard through the mid range of the exercise.

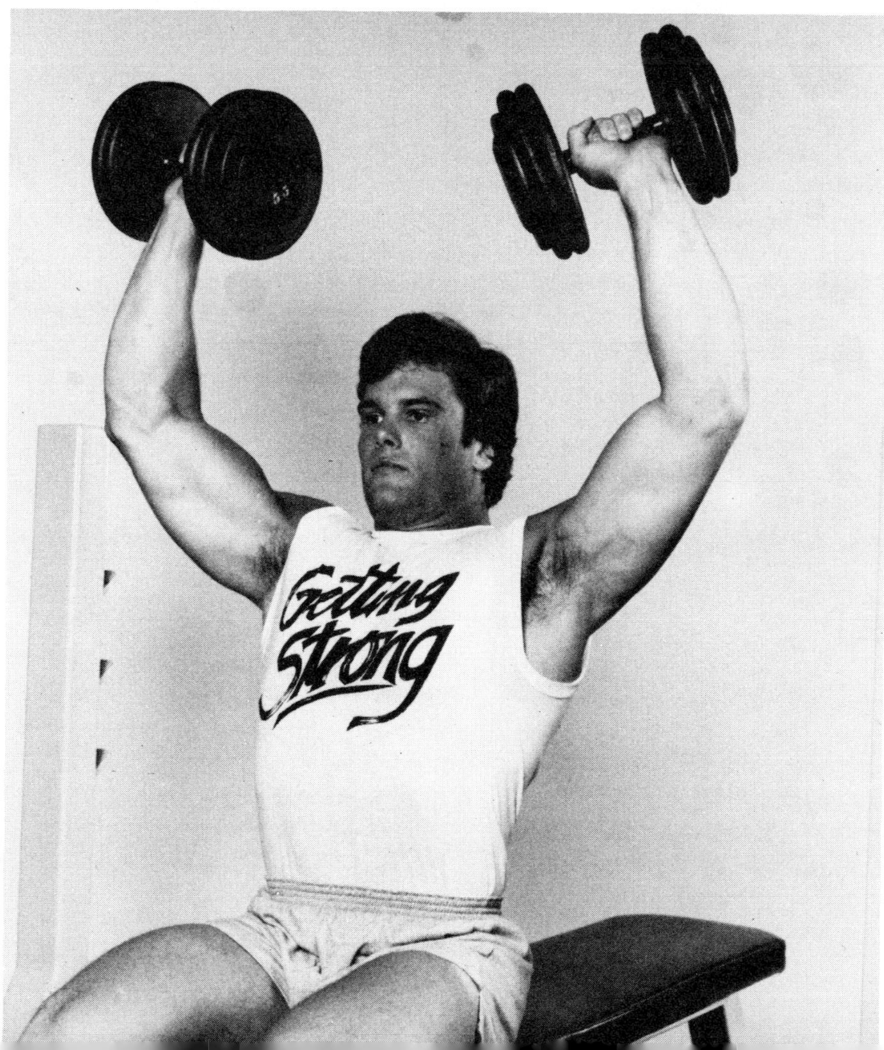

Your hands should come together as you near the completion of the Dumbbell Press. Good chest development must be complemented by a proportioned upper torso.

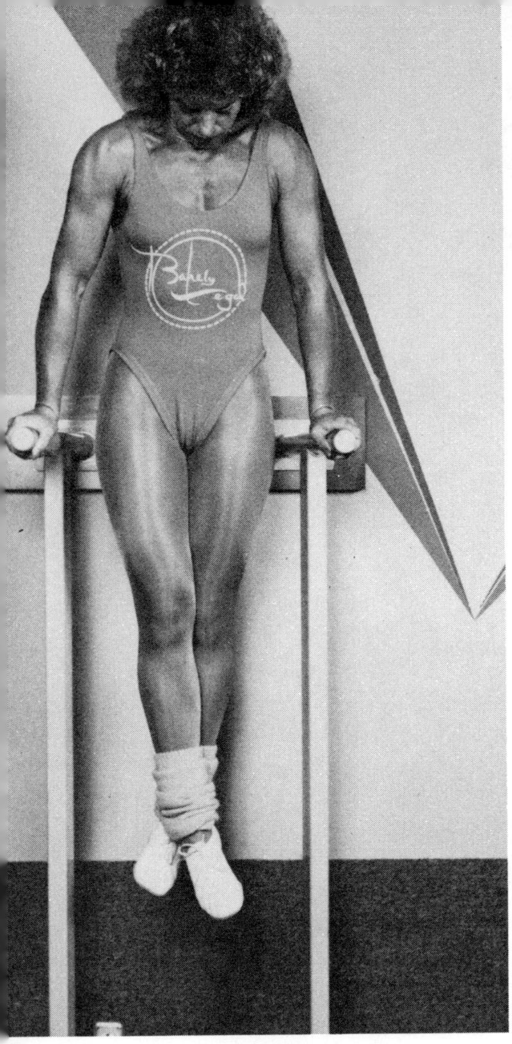

This is the starting position of the Parallel Bar Dip, demonstrated by Barbara Kline. The ankles should be crossed for increased stability during the movement.

◀

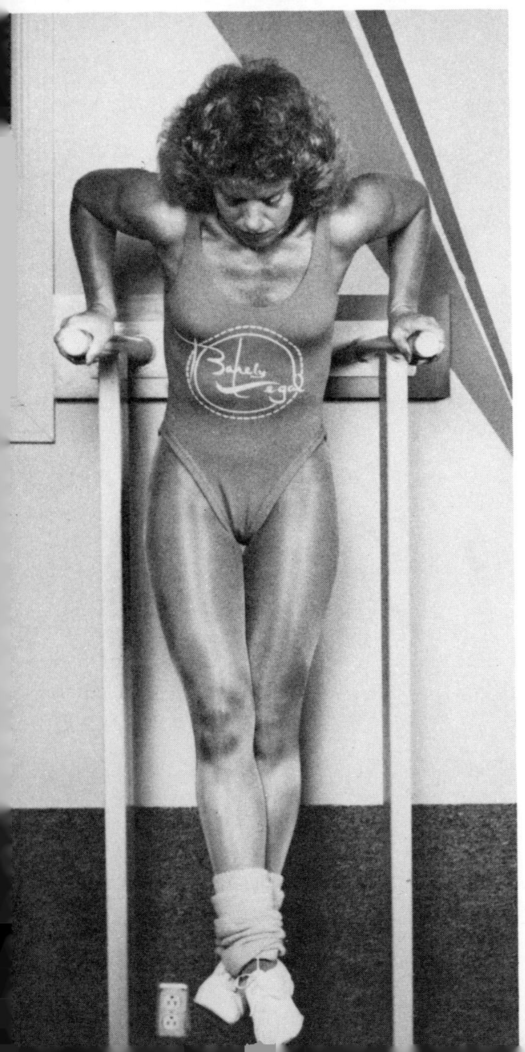

◀

At the stretched position of the Parallel Bar Dip, your shoulders should be lower than your elbows.

INTERMEDIATE BASIC CHEST ROUTINE

An intermediate bodybuilder trains four days a week on a split routine, working half the body on one day and the remaining half on the other. This lets you do more work for each body part without overtraining. The intermediate routine should still be slanted toward compound exercises, but isolation exercises to shape and build muscle are also included. Also, it is important for the intermediate to include exercises that stress the muscle on the length contraction (flyes) as well as the mid range (such as bench presses).

Barbell or Dumbbell Incline Press (alternate each workout),4 sets of 15, 12, 10, 8 reps. (Inverted pyramid, add weight each set.)

Flat Bench Barbell Press, 4 sets of 15, 12, 10, 8 reps. (Add weight each set.)

Flat or Incline Bench Fly 2-4 sets × 12-15 reps (same weight each set).

At this point the intermediate bodybuilder needs to focus on slow growing areas of the pecs and getting a strong pump in the muscles. Go as heavy as possible, but always use weights that allow you to feel the pecs throughout the full range of motion. On the flyes, work for the best burn possible, teaching yourself how to transcend the pain.

ADVANCED BASIC CHEST ROUTINE

Advanced bodybuilders are now training on a three-day on, one day off cycle, which allows them to train and deplete the entire body before giving it a day of rest. Some advanced trainers go six days straight.

More isolation exercises are done at the advanced level, corresponding to the weak point(s) of the chest. Mid-range contraction exercises (presses), length contraction exercises (flyes) and peak contraction exercises (pec dec) should always be included. Because of the heavy weights involved, the triceps can give out rapidly if you follow one movement with another. Instead, alternate an isolation exercise with a basic exercise. Advanced bodybuilders need to change the order and style of the exercises frequently to keep stimulated. Alternate dumbbell, barbell and cable variations for the exercises listed as desired, but leave the basic structure intact.

	Reps per Set
45-degree Incline Press (dumbbell or barbell)	15, 12, 10, 8, 6, (add weight each set)
Flat Bench Fly (dumbbell or cable)	12-15 for 5 sets
10-degree Bench Press (dumbbell or barbell)	15, 12, 10, 8, 6
Pec Dec	12-15 for 5 sets

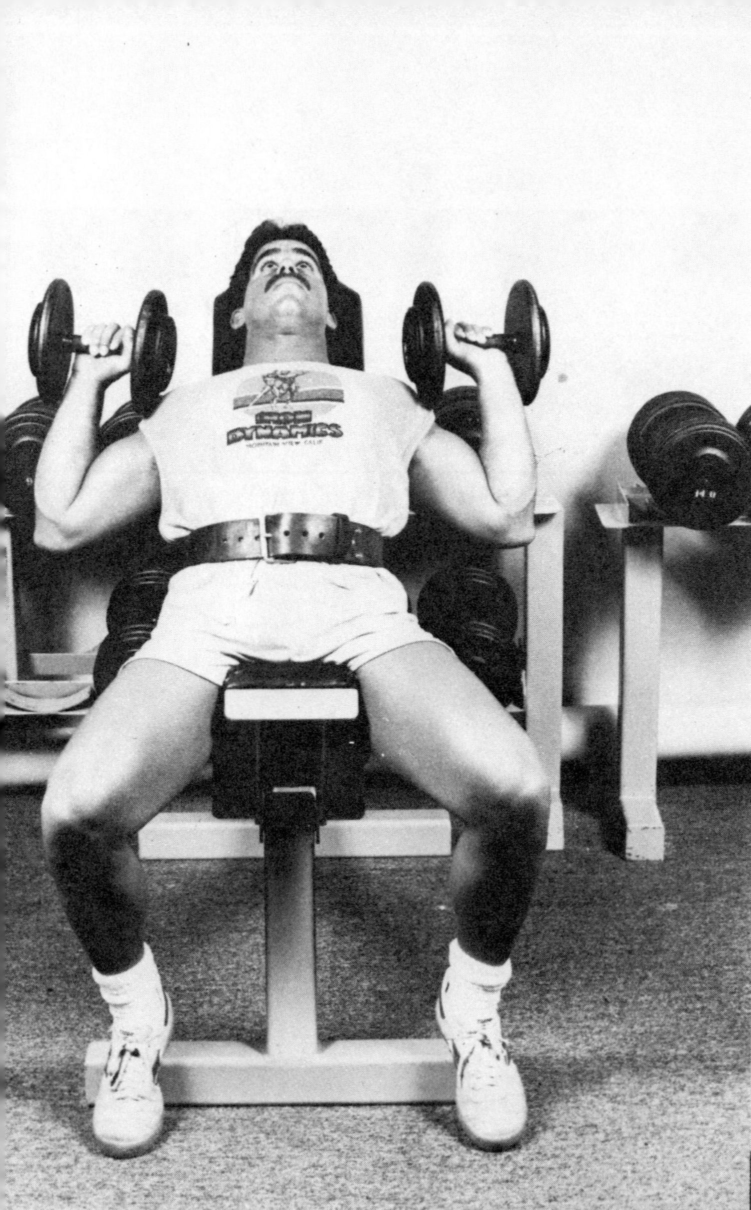

Your hands should come together at the completion of the Dumbbell Incline Press for maximum muscular contraction.

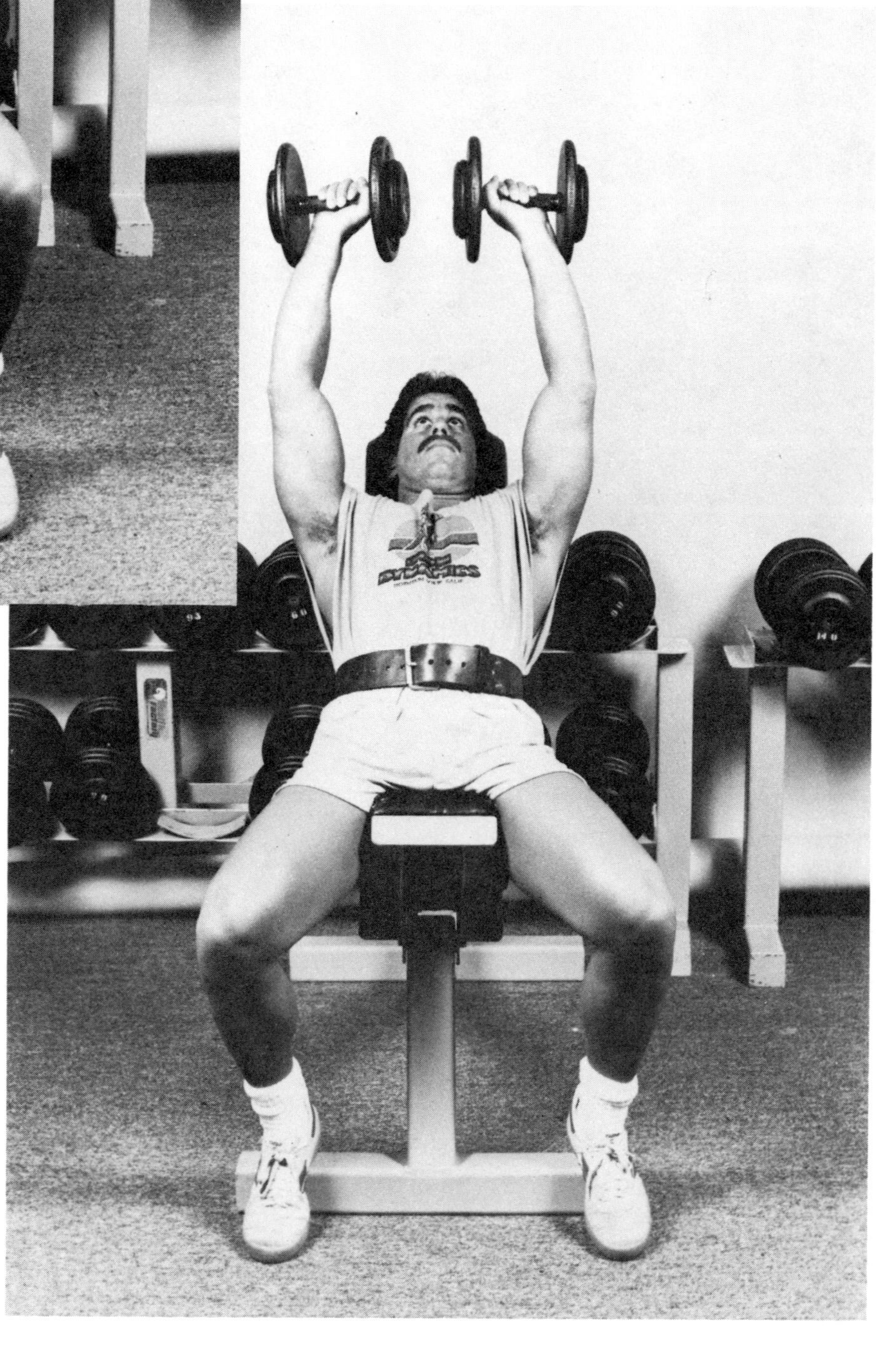

As with the Dumbbell Shoulder Press, Incline Dumbbell Presses are performed with your elbows out and to the sides.

This routine provides all the stimulation needed for advanced gains by varying the repetition schemes from strength (inverted pyramid) reps to endurance (straight sets of 15) reps. The muscle is worked from a wide variety of angles and the routine can be varied frequently without changing the basic structure.

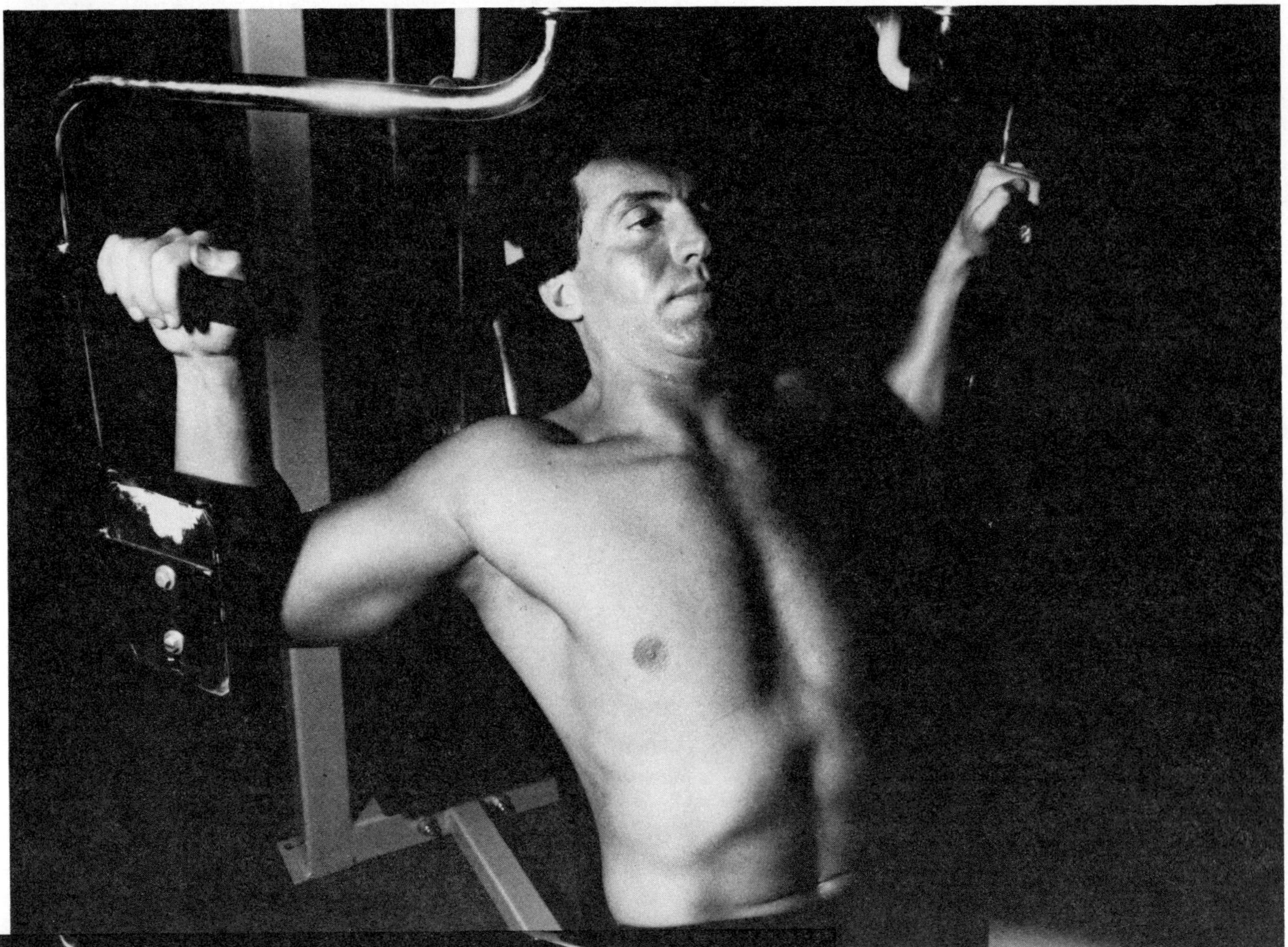

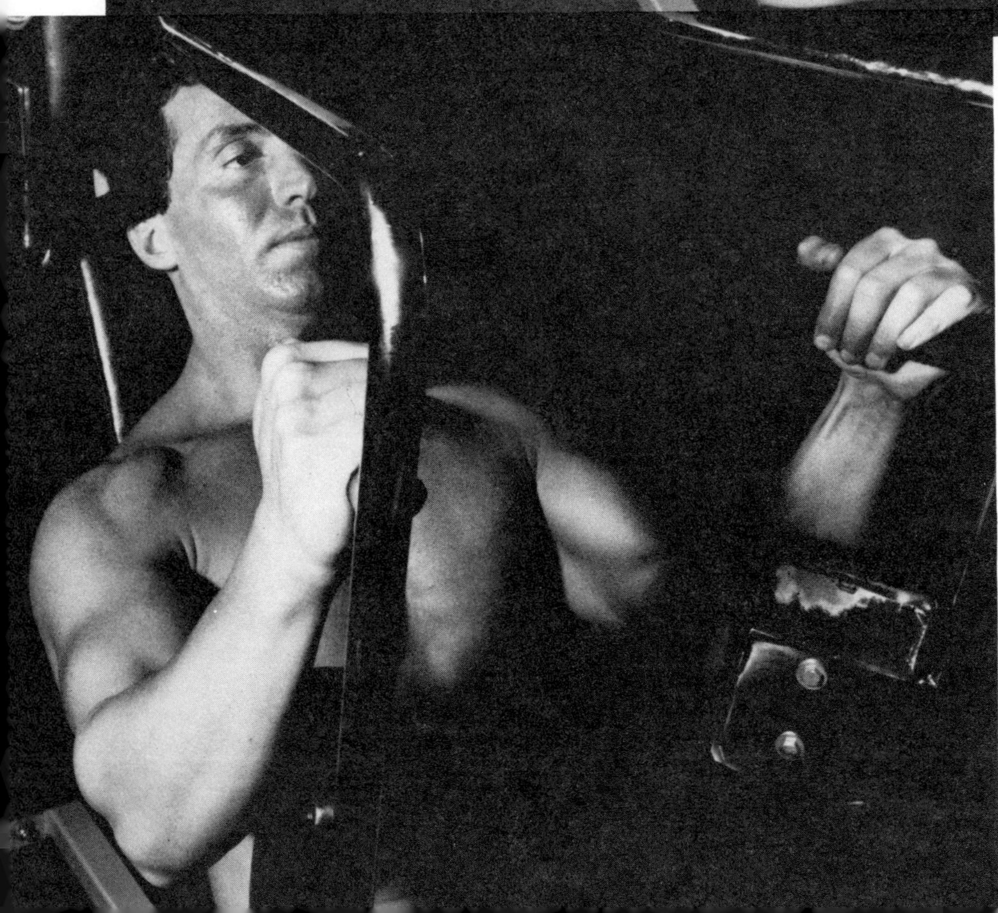

▲

Chest machines provide resistance throughout a full range of motion, putting maximum emphasis on the center or cleavage of the chest. Ray Vakili demonstrates the stretched position of this exercise.

◀ *Force should be applied with the elbows when using the pec dec chest machine. Some people go so far as to keep their palms open during the movement to avoid the tendency to apply force with the hands and upper arms.*

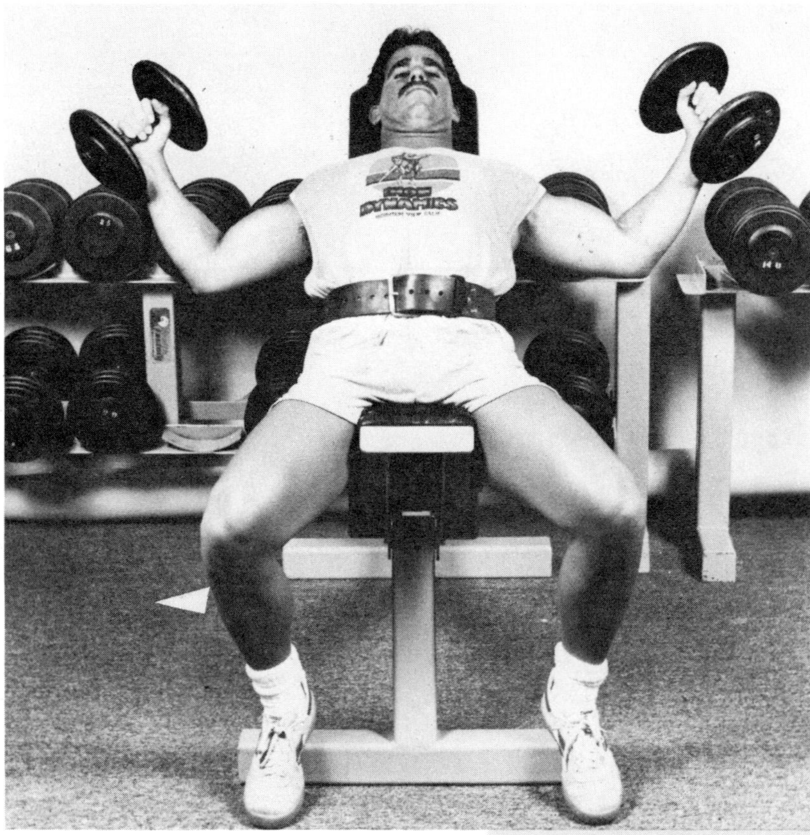

This is the stretched position of the Incline Dumbbell Bench Fly—one of the most essential upper chest developers. The upper arms should remain at right angles to the torso throughout the exercise.

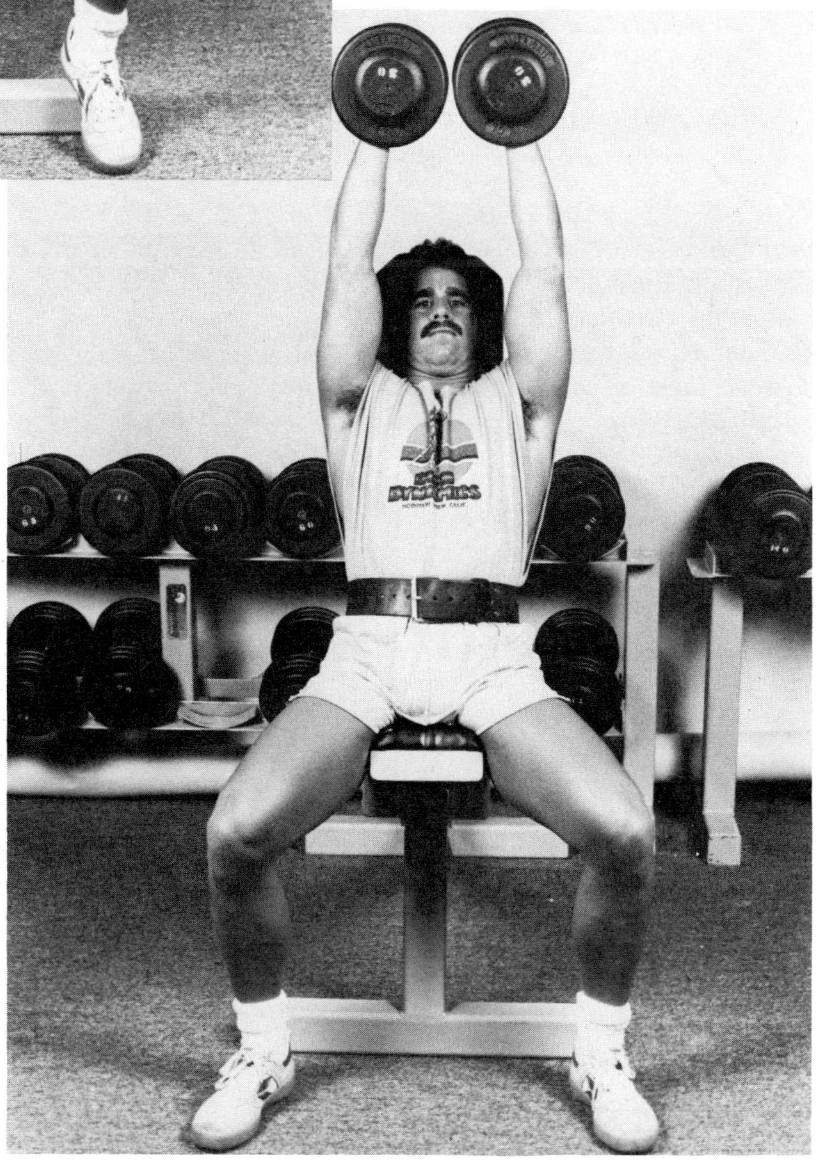

The edges of the dumbbells should touch at the completion of the dumbbell fly.

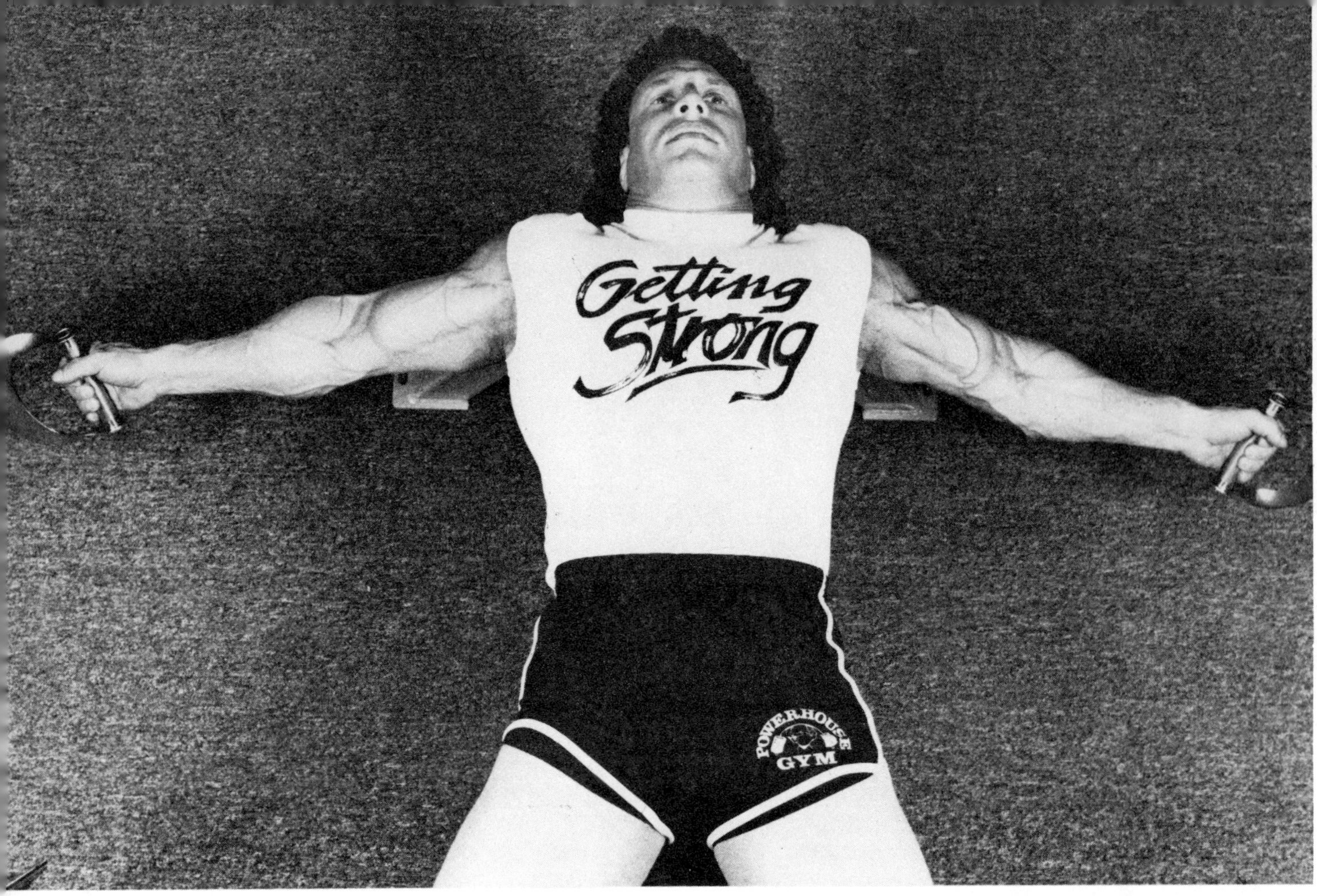

▲

Mr. America, Mr. Universe Don Ross demonstrates how to use cables in a fly movement to put maximum stress on the pectorals. Keep your elbows slightly unlocked to reduce the stress on the elbows.

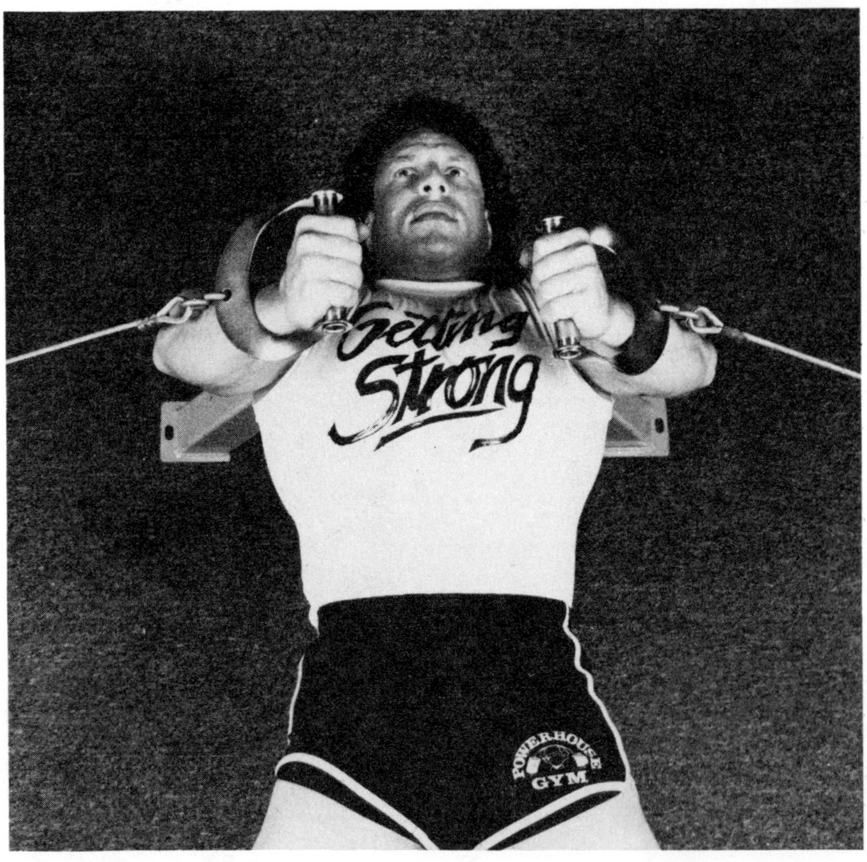

▶

Your hands should come together at the completion of the cable fly movement.

Chris Kiesman demonstrates proper form during the Bench Press. From this position the barbell is pressed straight up to the starting position to complete one repetition. ▶

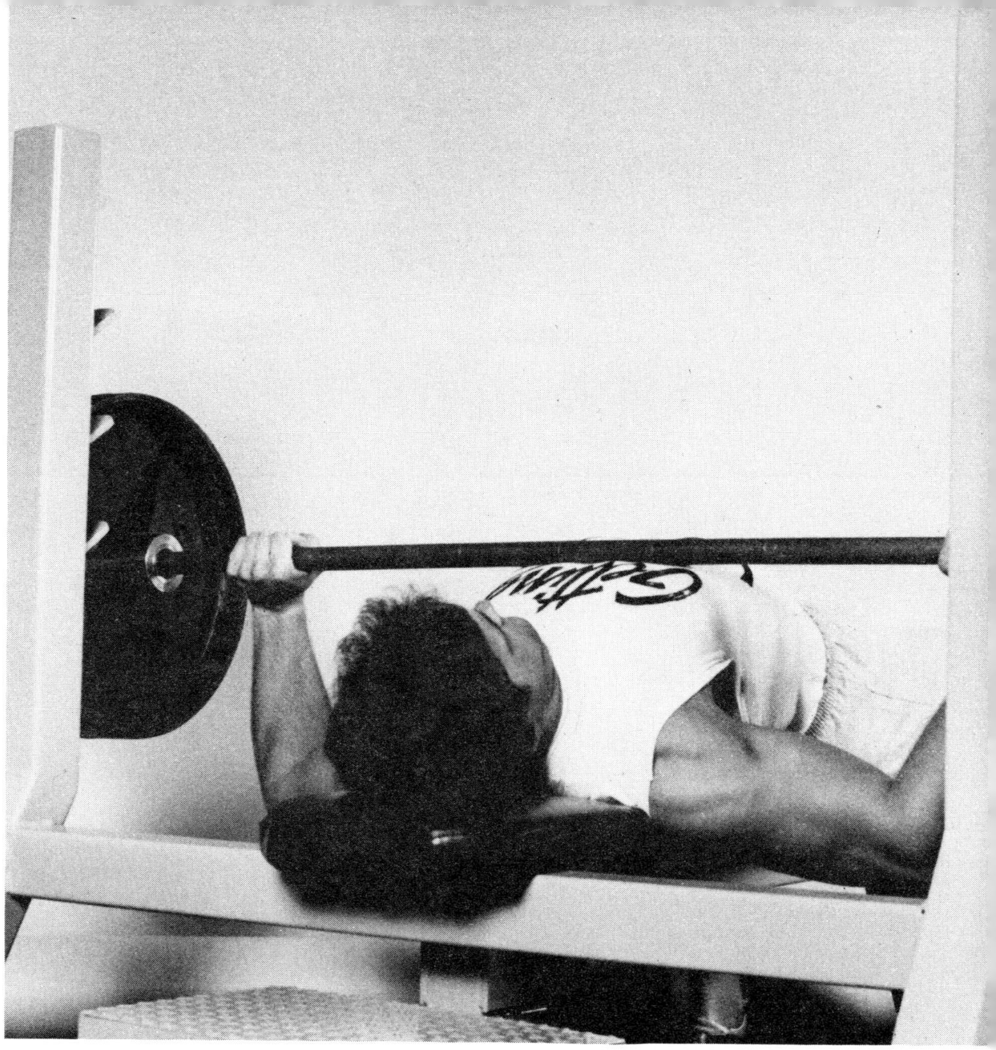

The Bench Press is the most popular chest exercise and one of the best upper-body strength developers. To avoid injury, do not lift your head or hips during the press.

▼

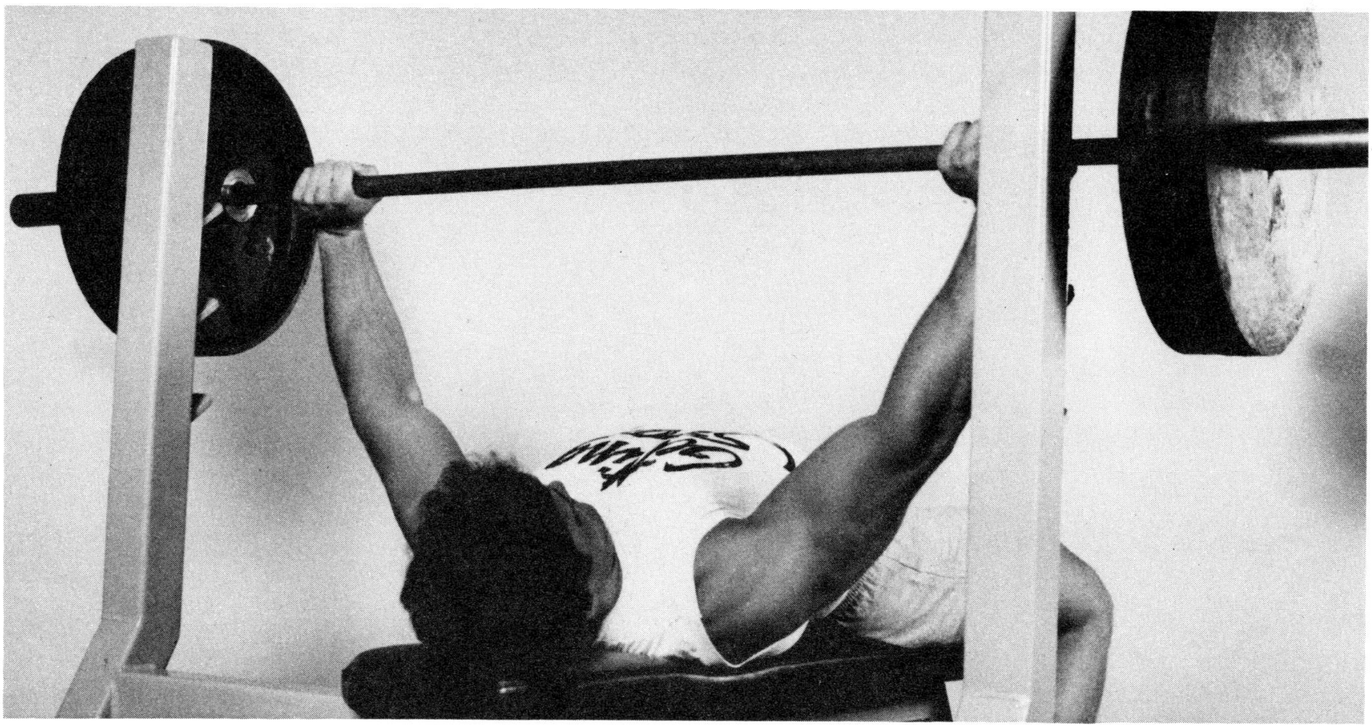

EIGHT: SIZE AND DENSITY

Gym tradition has it that low, heavy reps are done to increase size, and light pumping reps are used for better definition. This is not altogether accurate. All the sets that you do, no matter what the rep scheme, must be heavy and must overload if you want to stimulate adaptation. Low, heavy reps only work a different part of the cell than heavy high reps, causing a different result.

There is also a synergistic effect promoted by training all the cell components. Synergy is a principle that says that the whole has greater energy than the sum of its parts. In other words, training all cell components concurrently will produce a larger cell than what the sum of training each component separately would produce. This is scientifically sound because as the components grow, the surrounding cellular fluid, the sarcoplasm, increases in volume to accommodate the new, larger cell components.

Since each cell organelle has its own function, it will take a diversity of loads and intensity levels to induce an adaptation again. Overloading the muscle with low, medium and high repetitions, as well as varying the tempo and rhythm of the reps, is the core of size training.

Each repetition affects a different part of the cell. Training with low reps (four to six) and high intensity (85 percent or greater of max weight) stimulates the basic myofibril muscle fiber to grow thicker, larger and have more contractile force. It also increases muscle density by increasing the amount of cellular proteins it stores. Connective tissue strength and joint strength are stressed by reps in this range. In order to guarantee stimulation, the work must overload the muscle and ask it to work at its maximum for a specific number of reps.

Strength training with low reps is the foundation for size training. Training for low-rep strength enhances strength in your reps across the board. Being able to bench 315 pounds for six reps will make 225 pounds for 12 reps or more quite easy.

Medium reps (6 to 15) will stimulate a hypertrophy adaptation of the same basic muscle fiber. This is usually the rep range most advanced bodybuilders end up using, and if any one rep scheme is going to be done exclusively, this one would be the best choice. Fortunately you now know the consequences of training only one part of the muscle cell: never reaching your ultimate size potential.

High and heavy reps are also important to size training. The capillary and mitochondria systems of the cell increase both in size and number in response to high, overload reps. Blood flow to the muscles is increased, making for a more

Lori Bowen-Rice, 1984 winner of the professional women's World Championships, hits a side chest pose that clearly shows why she is one of the best.

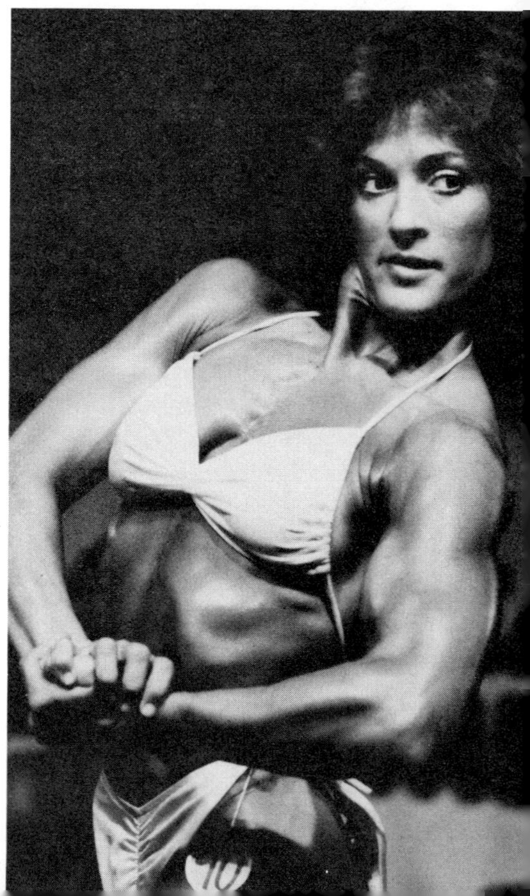

efficient circulatory system, essential if you are going for massiveness. Huge muscle mass without the circulation to supply it with blood and remove waste products is setting the stage for a training injury.

The endurance systems of the muscles make up to 30 percent of cell size. If you don't consistently train overload high reps, you are missing out on a third of the mass you could have. High rep training really makes everything else seem so much easier. After sets of 15 in the Bench Press, doing any exercise for only six reps seems too easy.

Basic compound exercises stimulate the most mass and stress the large belly of the muscle through the mid range. These are exercises such as Barbell and Dumbbell Bench Presses (on a flat, incline or decline bench). Variety is still required to keep the CNS and muscles stimulated, which is accomplished through changing style or grip rather than exercises.

Although size is your goal, arrange your basic size exercises to coincide with proportion goals, unless you are a rank beginner. Beginners need to learn to bench.

If you have never included power training in your routine, even though you have decent pec mass and shape, you might benefit from a month or two of power chest training. It will increase the strength in all your isolation exercises, give you more confidence and give your entire upper body a strength and size boost.

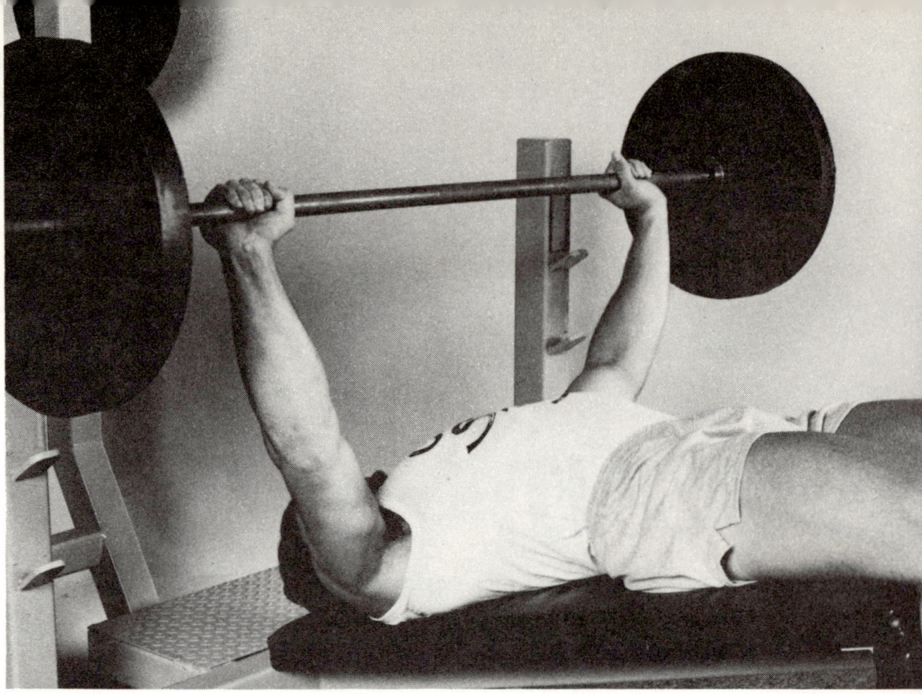

▲

Pictured is the starting position for the Decline Bench Press, an excellent exercise for the lower pecs.

As with the traditional Bench Press, the bar is lowered to the chest during this declined version of the press.

▼

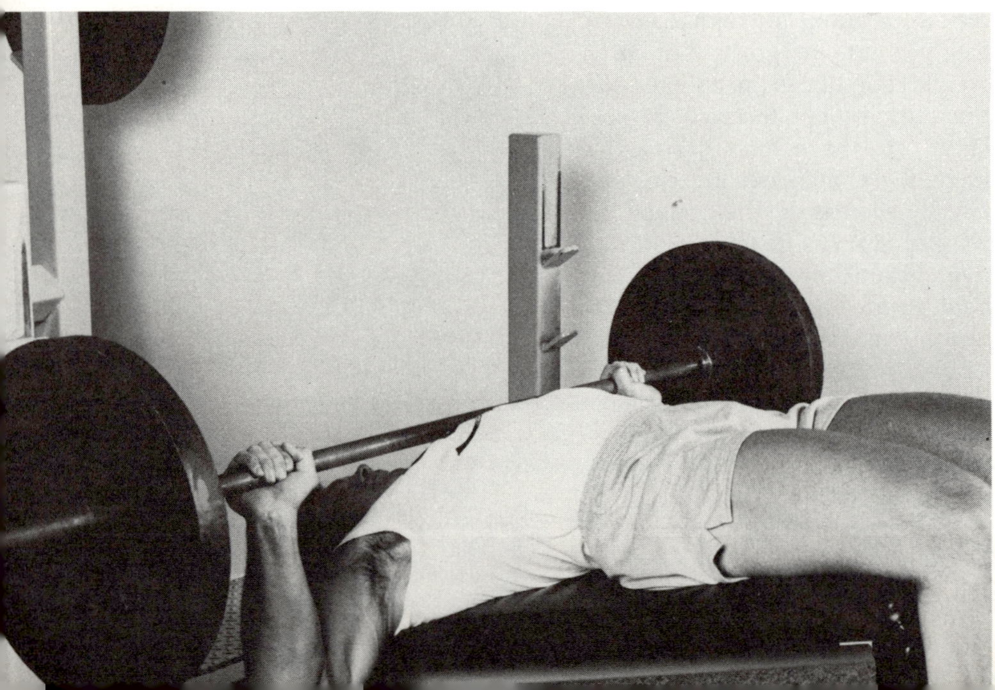

Training for size involves a variety of exercises and repetition schemes, but mostly it involves obtaining a power mentality. Your form must be perfect, and the movements as heavy and as powerful as possible. Always lower rather than drop the weights and be as explosive as possible on the positive rep.

SIZE ROUTINES

Inverted Pyramid Basic Size Routine

This is the most basic size routine utilizing the Bench Press, Dips and Flat Bench Flyes. Each of the exercises uses the inverted pyramid rep scheme so that all the muscle fiber gets exposed to the various rep stresses.

Begin the routine with the power Bench Press with a shoulder-width grip. Lower the bar to the middle of the pecs. Start with 15 reps and add weight each set, going for 12, 10, 8 6. Don't add weight unless you get all the reps.

Next go to weighted Dips, again using the inverted pyramid rep scheme. This lets you warm up safely to very heavy reps. Use the

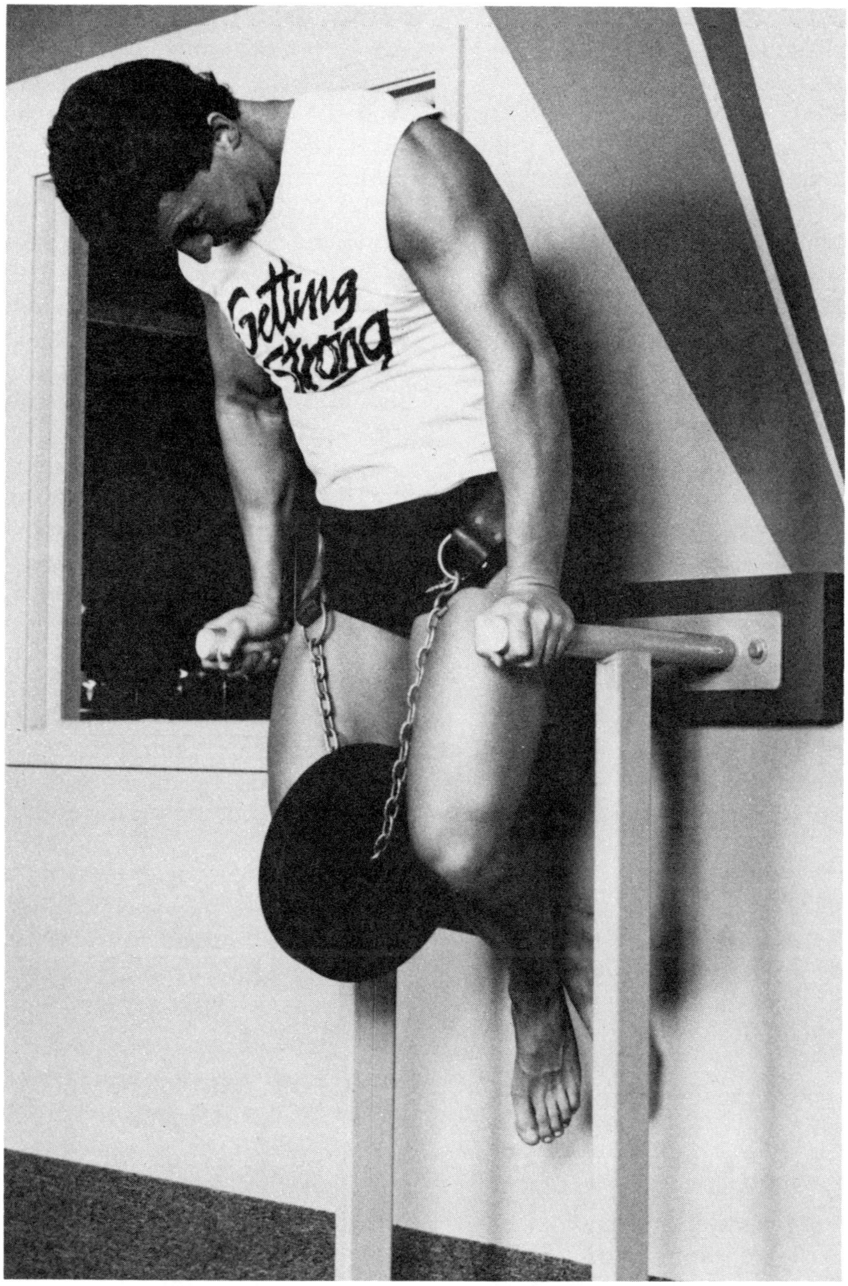

To increase the difficulty of bar dips, you can attach a plate to a dipping belt.

Here is the stretched position of the Bar Dip with Weights.

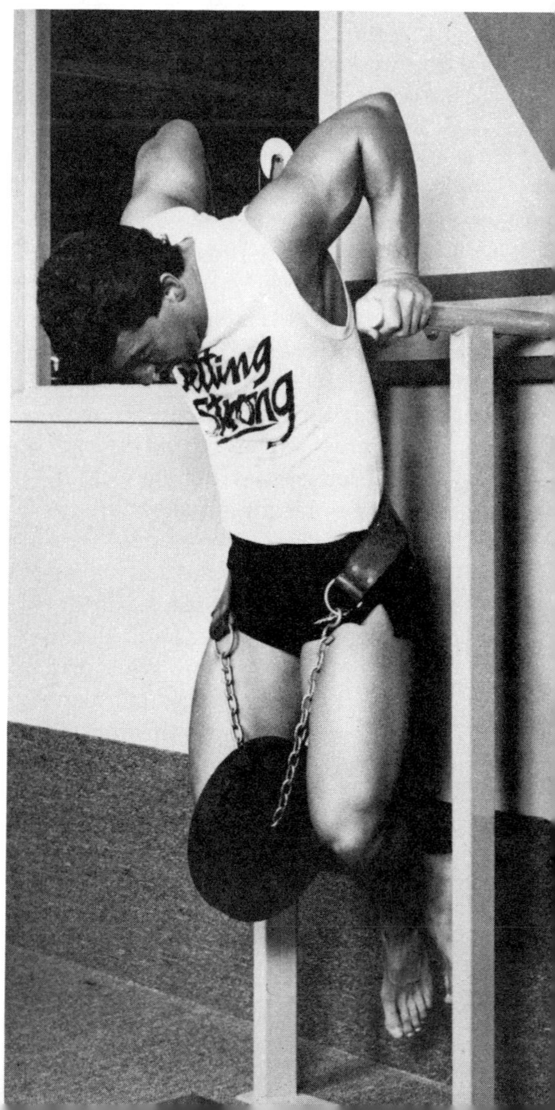

power Dip position, lowering with the back round and chin on the chest, but blast out of the bottom with triceps power. In using explosive movements, it is essential to never break form. If you do, you will eventually be injured. Never use weights that you cannot control.

Go next to Flat Bench Flyes, focusing on the length contraction (stretch) and keeping the arms locked in the semi-bent position. Keep the dumbbells parallel at all times. Keeping the upper back arched and the torso rotated up concentrates the stress on the pecs. Do five sets, inverted pyramid style, 15-6.

	Reps per Set
Flat Bench Barbell Bench Press	15, 12, 10, 8, 6
Weighted Dip	15-6 for 5 sets
Flat Bench Fly	15-6 for 5 sets

Inverted Pyramid Barbell Compound Exercise Routine

By utilizing only compound pressing exercises, you can expose the pecs, delts and triceps to very heavy workloads with the stability of the barbell. Even when fatigued from many sets of pressing, you will be able to use heavier weights than if you did the same exercises with dumbbells.

Start with Barbell Bench Presses with a shoulder-width grip, do five sets and increase the weight, dropping reps each set. Remember to keep the body as tight as possible for those heavy reps.

Go to Barbell Incline Presses with a close grip, working the upper inner pecs, a very important and hard-to-reach area. The close grip will also blow up the triceps. Don't worry about saving their strength as the next exercise is the Wide-Grip Decline Press with a barbell. Using a 30-degree decline bench, bring the bar down to the lower pec line and focus on contracting the lower pecs.

Barbell Bench Press 6×15, add weight each set, medium grip

Barbell Incline Press 6×15, add weight, close grip

Barbell Decline Press 6×15, wide grip

This is a very difficult routine. Don't expect your poundages to be very high by the time you get to the declines. It will take all the strength and energy you have to get through this routine even with light weight. The key is hitting all aspects—upper, middle and lower—pecs with three sets of each of the various rep schemes. This provides maximum stimulation for all areas and all cell components. I use the wide grip because by this time your triceps will be tired out. Train this routine only once a week.

Power Fives

Powerlifters, who nobody accuses of being small, like sets of five in the off-season for developing functional strength, density and mass. It's these high-intensity reps that increase the packing ratio of the cellular proteins and create that thick muscle tissue. Free cycle this workout, or use the heaviest weight for each set of five, taking one and a half minutes rest between sets; change the weight as necessary to get the reps.

Utilize a power bench position on the Bench Press and a palms-forward position with the dumbbells. This brings the shoulders into the action, making a less isolated but stronger press.

Medium-Grip Barbell Bench Press 5×5

Incline Dumbbell Press 5×5

This routine works the bench extremely heavy and the Incline Presses help keep the surrounding stabilizers strong through the full range of motions the dumbbells travel and the inherent instability of the dumbbells.

Power Bench and Assistance Exercise Routine

When training exclusively for muscle hypertrophy you should avoid becoming "too efficient" in a movement, lest your muscle becomes so efficient it stops adapting. With power training you need your efficiency and technique to be at its best. Train for a "groove" on the bench with the same technique, but vary the style and technique of the assistance exercises to keep the muscles surrounding the area growing.

Start the routine with the Power Bench Press. Arch your upper back and plant your feet firmly for maximum body leverage. Do five sets of 10, 8, 6, 6, and 6 focusing on explosive positive reps and controlled negative reps. Do not bounce the bar off your chest. Each set should be a max effort, aiming for one max set of six.

Assistance exercises also strengthen the weak links in the lift. For triceps power and development, use Narrow-Grip Bench Presses with a straight or cambered bar, both hands one inch from the center of the bar. Lower the bar with the elbows tucked into the sides. The bar should be brought to the low pec line.

The 75-degree Dumbbell Press works the clavicle area of the pecs as well as the anterior deltoid, both of which help stabilize the shoulder girdle during a heavy bench. Keep the palms forward to maximize shoulder involvement and press to three-quarters lockout only.

Use body weight Dips to finish the triceps and pecs with a strong stretch and pump. Use a combination dipping motion, going down as if for chest (leaning forward, chin on chest, back round) and coming up using the triceps (elbows tucked in to sides).

Power Bench Press 4×10, 8, 6, 6, (working up to one max set of six)

Narrow-Grip Bench Press 4×6 (three-second pause on last rep of each set)

Seated 75-degree Dumbbell Press 5×8 (as heavy as possible, palms facing the head)

Body Weight Dip 4 sets maximum reps, including max negatives on last set

POST-EXHAUST SIZE TRAINING

This is the only super-set system I use, and a favorite. By doing the isolation exercise after the compound I can have both: use heavy poundages on my basic exercises and not rob them of their strength stimulation. I can also pump and burn the pecs with the Pec Decs right after and concentrate on the contraction, knowing I don't have to face a heavy, dangerous exercise in an already exhausted state.

Adjust the Pec Dec seat and keep your back flat against the pad. Focus on keeping the torso rotated upward (remember this position) and holding the peak contraction for two seconds, flexing against the resistance as much as possible. Make sure you get to this exercise immediately after the presses to take advantage of the pecs' weakened condition.

Dumbbell Bench Press (angle determined by priority need) 15×6, add weight each set

Pec Dec 5 sets of 12-15 reps, same weight; three to four super-sets

Power Dip Routine

As a gymnast I spent years working on the parallel bars and doing the dipping motion to get up and down from the bars, for conditioning and for a variety of competitive skills. As a result, my pecs were always my most developed and refined body part. My shoulders, triceps and rib cage also grew stronger and thicker from the full range stress.

The Dip is one of the best exercises for the torso because of the tremendous range of motion and the variety of contractions it generates. Done properly, dipping all the way down, chin on the chest and back rounded, it can give your physique or your benching strength a boost. With extra weight they can give you explosive upper body power and development.

Never drop or bounce out of the bottom position. Like squats and deadlifts, Dips give great results but there's a high risk of injury if done poorly or without concentration. Work into the full stretch position slowly, increasing your workable range of motion progressively.

Do the Power Dips with combination technique, going down with the back round, chin on the chest and hips bent at the waist to stretch the pecs, but drive through the positive part of the rep.

The Gironda Dips focus entirely on pec isolation by keeping the elbows out to the sides, chin down, back round. Using both these styles will give strength and shape to the chest and upper torso.

Parallel Bar Dip 15, 12, 10, 8, 6 (add weight each set)

Gironda Dip (chin on chest) 4-6 sets of max reps (body weight only)

I don't have tremendously long routines because I believe that if you work each set as it should be worked—with perfect form, intense contractions, a full range of motion and with the heaviest possible weights—you cannot do very many of them.

Strive for a perfect connection with the muscle and power through every inch of the range of motion. If there are parts of the rep that you cannot connect with, you are losing development in that area. Once you achieve this ability to connect the physical and mental, new bodybuilding vistas will unfold.

Capillary Pumping Size Routine

The basis of this routine is stressing the capillary system to its maximum to "plump" up the muscle cell. Vince Gironda says that although one is born and dies with the same number of muscle fibers (and cannot increase), one can obtain maximum shape by keeping the capillaries filled with blood. This works well, especially when you cannot, for whatever reason, train with heavier weights. The emphasis is on concentration training and isolation work for a good pump in the shortest amount of time.

Alternating isolation and compound exercises keeps the pecs working without the weaker triceps giving out too early. High-rep training drains less nervous energy than low-rep high-intensity training, and the routine can be done often, two times per week or three times in 10 days.

Start with Low Incline (30 to 40 degrees) Dumbbell Flyes to isolate the upper pecs. Total stretch is the key to intense flyes. Vary the angle of the incline as often as you desire and do four sets of 12 reps using the same weight for all four sets. Work hard and fast for a burn and pump.

Next go to Shoulder-Width Barbell Presses lowered to the mid-pec line (between nipple and throat), again going for four sets of 12 and only using as much weight on the bar as is comfortable.

Return to an isolation exercise: Decline Flyes to work the lower pecs. Concentrate on lowering the dumbbells as far back as possible; turn the palms slightly forward on the descent and return them back to parallel on the positive part of the rep. This really isolates the lower pecs. Do four sets of 12.

Finish the pump with high-rep Shoulder-Width Push-ups, stopping just shy of lockout. Do as many reps as possible each set, two to four sets.

	Sets	Reps
Incline Dumbbell Fly	4	12
Medium-Grip Barbell Flat Bench Press	4	12
Decline Dumbbell Fly	4	12
Shoulder-Width Push-up	2-4	max

Serge Nubret Pro Rep System

This workout is similar to capillary pumping except that it is progressive. Instead of increasing the weight each set, Nubret increases the reps! This is not easy, no matter what weight is used. He also strives to keep the rest periods as short as possible, bringing a good supply of blood to the muscle. This is an excellent system for those who respond better to high reps or cannot go heavy.

Nubret uses basic exercises and total concentration. Begin the workout with non-lockout Barbell Bench Presses, bringing the bar to the throat. Use a wide grip. Start each exercise with 10 reps and add two reps each set, finishing with five sets and 18 reps on the last set.

Go next to Wide-Grip Incline Barbell Presses with the same rep scheme, again to the throat with non-lockout reps. Finish the routine with Flat Bench Flyes for five sets of progressive reps. The pump and burn in this routine is right up there with the best. It is good in the beginning of a cycle when volume and low-intensity work is called for. The high reps develop a superior circulatory system and strengthen the joints.

Wide-Grip Bench Press (non-lock) 5×10, 12, 14, 16, 18 (same weight each set)

Wide-Grip Incline Barbell Press 5×10, 12, 14, 16, 18

Flat Bench Fly 5×10, 12, 14, 16, 18

MULTI-CONTRACTION SIZE TRAINING

Multi-contraction size training involves doing length, peak and mid-range contractions, each with a varying repetition scheme. The workout exposes all the muscle fibers to the full variety of different rep scheme stresses. By doing a length contraction exercise, a peak contraction exercise and a mid-range contraction exercise, you work the fibers in all their capacities.

The exercises are: Incline (45-degree) Dumbbell Flyes, for the length contraction, Pec Dec, for the peak contraction, and the Barbell Bench Press for the heavy, mid-range contraction. Organize the workout by starting with the most needed exercise.

If your inner pecs are the weakest, start with the Pec Dec; if upper pecs are what you need most, begin with Incline Flyes. Starting with flat benches will give the belly of the pecs the heaviest stress first.

Focus on stretching the flyes to the maximum, holding the peak contraction of the Pec Dec for two seconds. By simultaneously stimulating all areas of the muscle with the various types of contractions, the pecs will respond very quickly. For each exercise do either four sets of five, four sets of 10 or four sets of 15.

Keeping the rep ranges far apart ensures that different cell mechanisms are being stressed. Start with one exercise and one rep scheme and do that for a week or two, then rotate the reps to different exercises.

For example:

WEEK ONE

Incline Dumbbell Fly	4×5
Pec Dec	4×10
Barbell Bench Press	

WEEK TWO

Incline Dumbbell Fly	4×10
Pec Dec	4×15
Barbell Bench Press	4×5

You can vary the exercise order, unless you have a serious weak point that demands doing a specific exercise first, when your energy is highest.

MID-PEC THICKNESS AND SIZE ROUTINE

Very often the hardest area to gain size in is the inner and central pecs. This is especially true if you do most of your chest training with a wide grip. Contrary to tradition, wide-grip benches do not stretch the pecs maximally. Wide-grip benches mainly stress the outer section of the pecs. The result can be wide pecs, but it will not give mid-pec thickness or size. For that you need to press with a shoulder-width grip and mid-range contraction exercises to stress the belly of the central pecs.

Use the Barbell Bench Press and a shoulder-width grip for five sets and work down from 15-6 reps. Bring the bar down to the mid-pec line and get as much stress as possible. If you have access to a cambered bar, use that. Next, go to Dumbbell Pullovers, tilting the dumbbell forward and pulling the shoulders together to get the inner pecs. Do four sets of 10 for a hypertrophy response. Finish the mid-pecs with Flat Bench Dumbbell Presses, palms facing each other throughout the exercise for four sets of five.

Barbell Flat Bench Press 5 sets of 15-6 reps, (inverted pyramid)

Tilting Dumbbell Pullover 4×10 reps

Flat Bench Dumbbell Press 4×5 reps

POWER DUMBBELL SIZE ROUTINE

Just as compound exercises with barbells stimulate well because of the heavy weight that can be involved, compound exercises with dumbbells also can be excellent for size training.

It's the perfect alternate routine for a barbell compound routine. You cannot handle as much total weight with dumbbells, but the increase in length contraction and range of motion more than compensates for the weight.

Many athletes find that heavy barbell exercises bother their shoulders after a while. The free rotational path dumbbells take removes a lot of stress from the joints.

Start the routine with Flat Bench Dumbbell Presses. Utilize a twisting motion to take full advantage of the dumbbells. Turn palms in on the negative rep and palms away on the positive rep. You get maximal stretch when you need it, as well as additional pressing power from the shoulders when it's needed. Do the basic size rep scheme, for five sets of 15-6 reps.

Go next to Incline Dumbbell Presses on a low incline bench (20 to 45 degrees). Use the same twisting action as on the Flat Dumbbell Benches with the same inverted pyramid rep scheme. Finish the pecs with Dumbbell Pullovers, tilting the dumbbell forward on the positive rep to engage the upper pecs. Again, do the five sets of 15-6 reps.

Flat Bench Twisting Dumbbell Press 5 sets of 15-6 reps

Low Incline Twisting Dumbbell Press 5 sets of 15-6 reps

Cross Bench Dumbbell Pullover 5 sets of 15-6 reps

REST BETWEEN SETS FOR MAXIMUM MUSCLE SIZE

For natural bodybuilders to obtain maximum muscle size, I believe it is essential to train for strength. Bodybuilders using

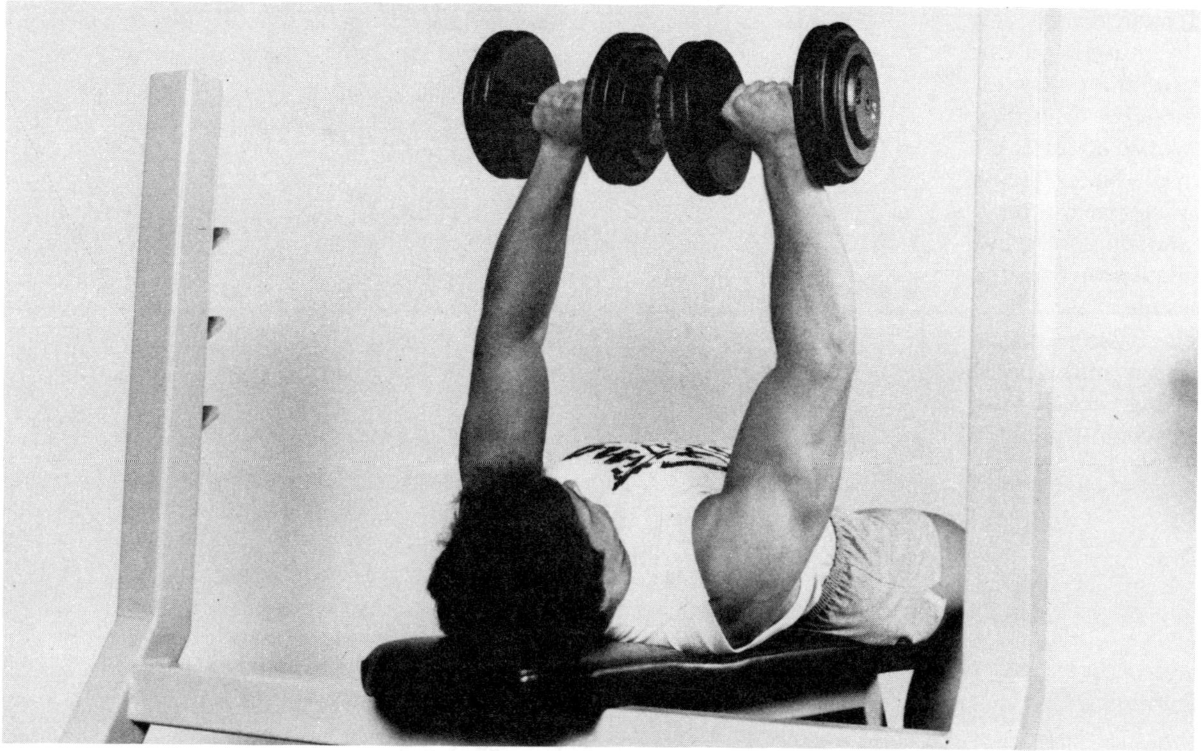

The Bench Press can also be performed with dumbbells. This is the start of the Flat Bench Twisting Dumbbell Press.

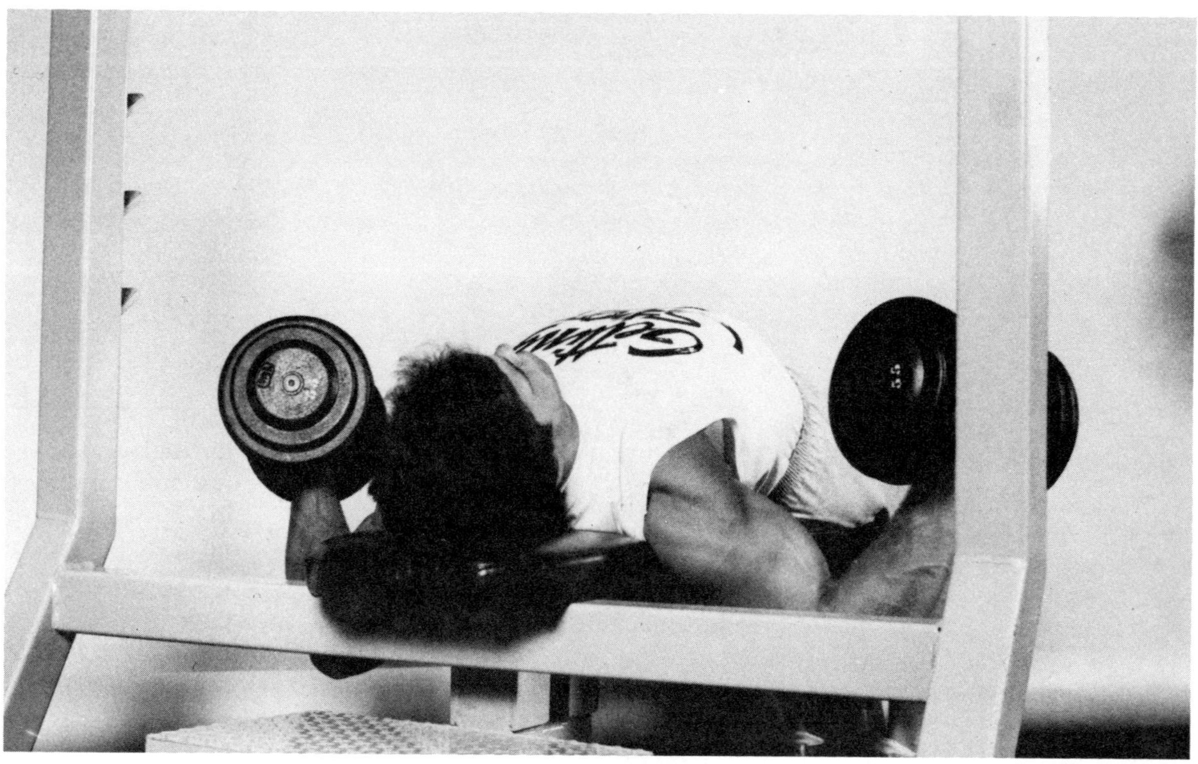

Dumbbell presses work the chest throughout a fuller range of motion than barbell presses, and the dumbbells also require the use of additional stabilizing muscles, which gives you a fuller development.

drugs to speed recuperation can "break down" muscle tissue through lighter weights and endless high-rep sets because they don't need to worry about overtraining. Natural bodybuilders cannot exceed very narrow recuperation limits and hope to grow. They must stimulate growth in the shortest time possible.

Hence, I believe basic exercises, and the inverted pyramid, are essential for getting big pecs. To train with the heaviest weights possible

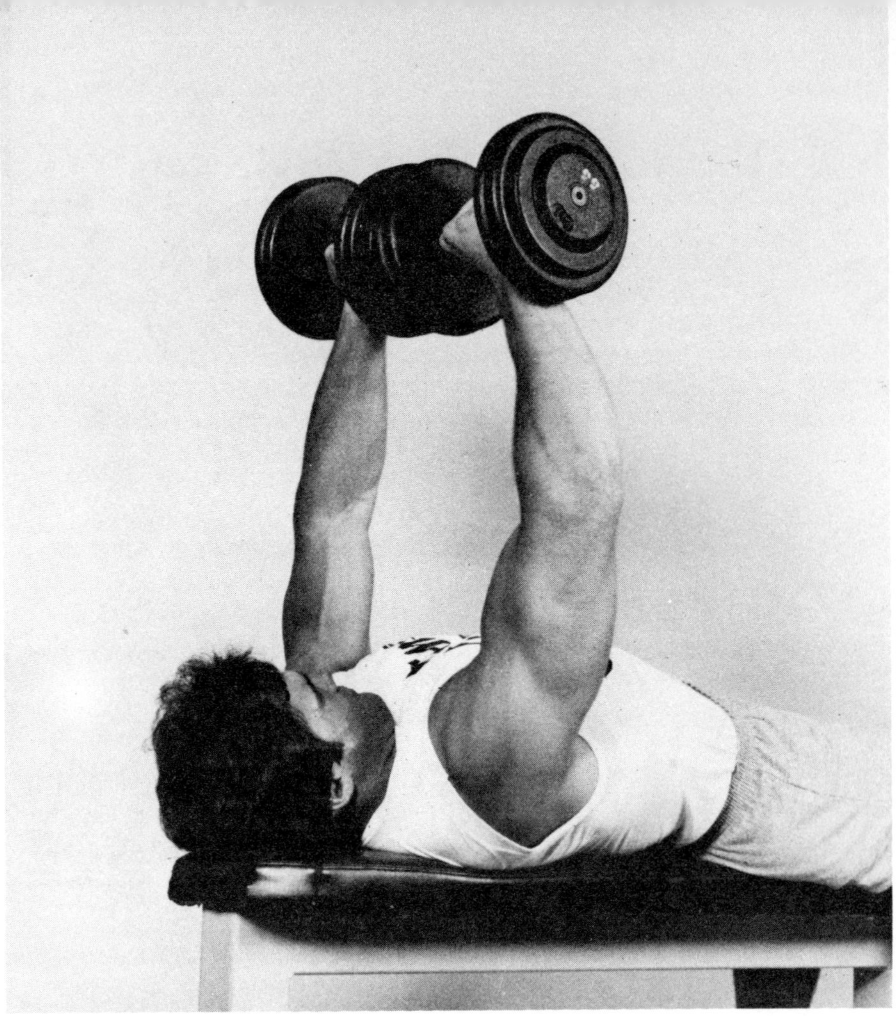

Increasing the angle of the bench during dumbbell presses shifts the emphasis on the muscle being worked. This is the starting position of Low Incline Twisting Dumbbell Press.

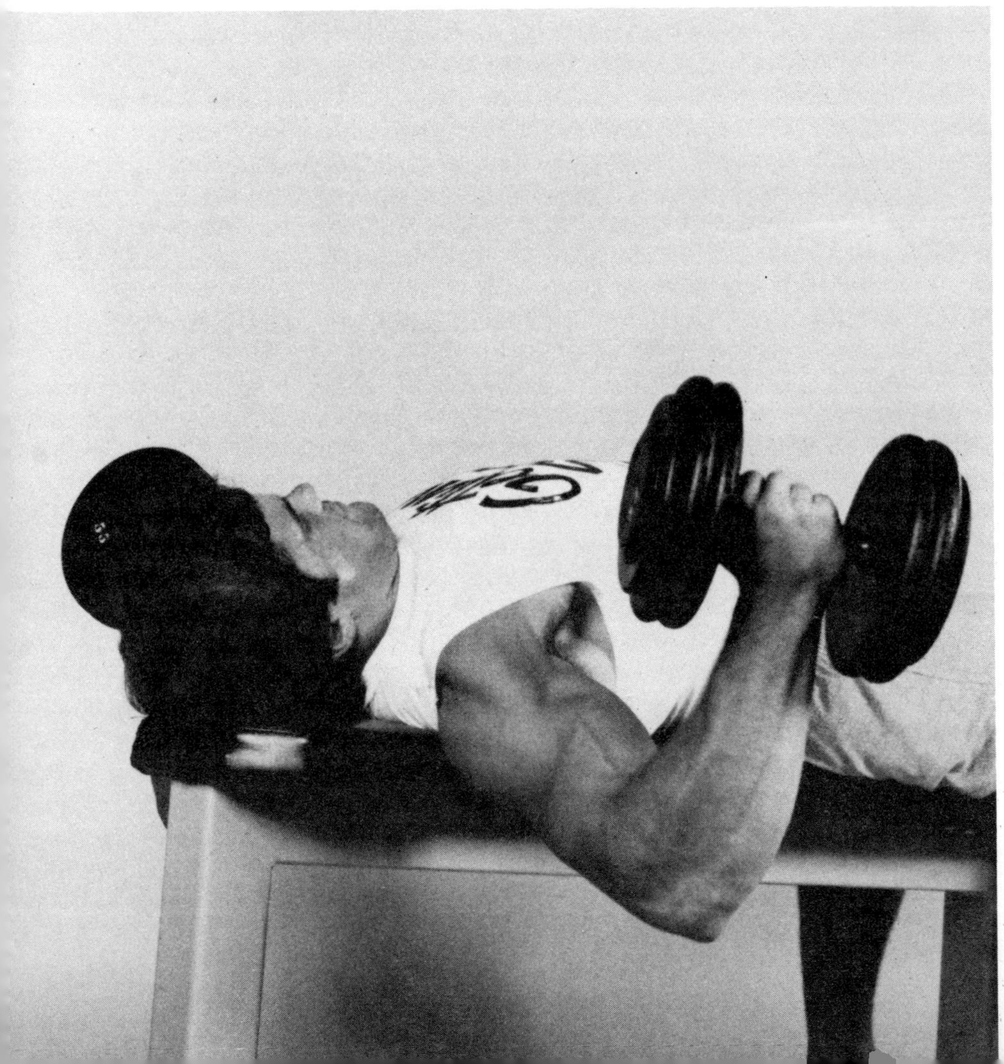

Chris Kiesman gets a full stretch as he finishes a twisting dumbbell press to add width and size on his chest.

for high and low reps, you must rest sufficiently between sets. Taking 30 seconds rest between sets negates the possibility of using heavy weights! If you are ready to go after only 30 seconds, that set didn't do too much to you.

Experiment with different rest times to see how long it takes to regain most of your strength. Different exercises will take more time than others. Train for strength and don't let your workout disintegrate into an aerobics class.

NINE: SHAPE AND SYMMETRY

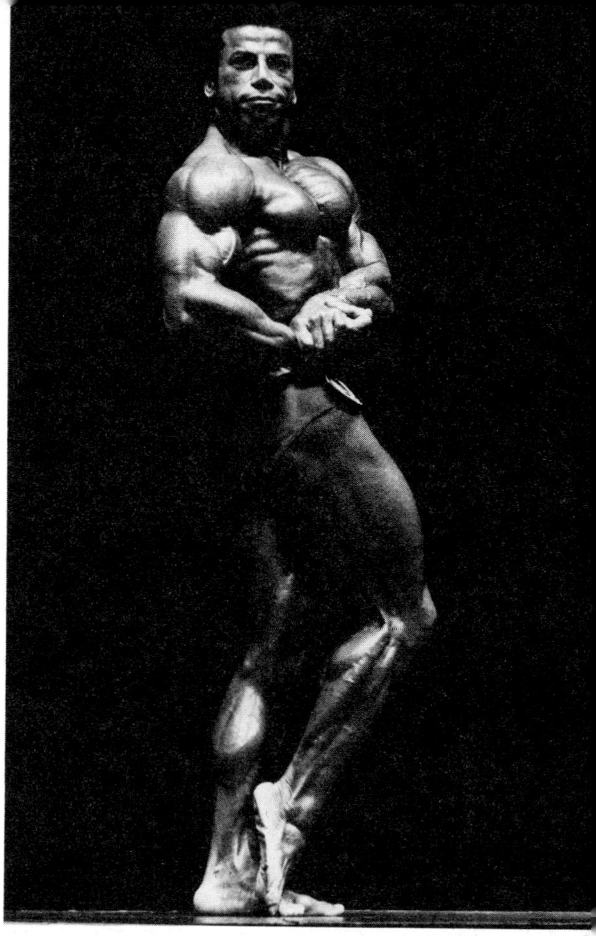

▲

Over 40 years old when he won the 1982 Mr. Olympia, Chris Dickerson is an inspiration to many people who begin bodybuilding in their later years.

Training the chest for shape and symmetry is one of the most rewarding tasks in bodybuilding. It is extremely challenging to design and do routines that change the look and shape of the chest.

Every body has different muscle lengths, inherent genetic shape and allocation of muscle cells and neurological abilities. Coupled with variations in hormonal levels, you have individuals with a muscle shape and frame that is totally unique to them. Instead of comparing yourself with others (especially "physique stars"), look at your strong and weak points and establish your routine to improve your shape and symmetry.

After you've been training awhile, you discover easy- and hard-gaining muscles. Your lower pecs might grow if you just look at the Bench Press, while your upper pecs may look as if they never touched an Incline Press. You must choose the appropriate routine to build aspects of the muscle that need the most work.

Muscle isolation goes along with training the areas that need the most work. When training for muscle shape, you must be able to isolate each area of the pecs from the others so that you can direct the tension accordingly.

Perfect form is a key to shape training. If you train your upper pecs, but arch so much that the bar gets lowered to the lower pecs, you are not working the upper pecs.

You must know what exercise with what form works what muscle section. In shape training, "feeling" the muscle contract over the range of motion is much more important than the weight on the bar. Usually the weight gets in the way of good contractions. You still need to be progressive with weight selection, but isolated muscle contractions with perfect form are a priority.

Use a different training tempo when shape training. No explosive power movement here! You need continuous tension through the full range of motion, length and peak contractions instead of the heavy mid-range contractions needed for size training and an emphasis on the negative rep.

Slightly higher reps work well with shape training, in the range of 10 to 15. Isolating the mid inner pec does not take heavy sets of six. It is much more delicate and refined work.

SHAPE TRAINING

If you have an area of your chest that is not growing, it could be because of poor muscle cell allocation to that area, which is genetically determined and cannot be changed. If you have very short muscles with long tendon attachments, the muscle will not be capable of growing to extremely large proportions.

Training for shape and capillary growth can plump up the cells and increase the illusion of size with a well-proportioned physique. A proportionate chest, such as Samir Bannout's or Mohammed Makkawy's, always looks impressive. The measurement that you could take would be irrelevant to the quality of the development. Many think shape training is the essence of bodybuilding. They may be right, as long as the public always chooses the shapely, proportionate and symmetrical bodybuilder over the huge but "uncut" version of the bodybuilder's physique.

Muscle isolation. If you cannot feel the individual muscle working, it is not working to its maximum. Strive to make the mind/body link as strong as possible. The stronger the mental involvement, the stronger the contraction. Through biofeedback techniques, people have learned how to fire single motor neurons within a muscle.

The smaller the area a bodybuilder directs his consciousness into, the stronger the neurological impulse into the area to activate the muscle. Being able to contract such small sections of the muscles allows you to completely control the shaping process, adding where you want it and leaving it alone where it's all right.

Length contraction. Length contraction exercises, such as flyes and pullovers, work the muscle most directly in the stretched position. The most productive part of any fly movement is the bottom when the arms act as levers and the chest is the fulcrum—all the tension is on the pecs. This is a specific type of contraction and has a unique shaping effect on the pecs when done regularly.

Bodybuilders who only do pressing movements for the pecs often look "bunched up" and tight. Flyes stretch out the muscle, making it look longer and more fluid. Stretching exercises also separate the various pectoral muscles with deep grooves, making their shape more apparent.

Peak contraction. The most growth stimulation occurs when the muscles are fully contracted. Most exercises provide little or no resistance in this very important position. When the resistance is direct, as in a Pec Dec or Cable Crossover, the maximum number of motor units and muscle fibers are forced into use, creating a very strong and productive contraction. Peak contraction exercises for the chest thicken, striate and add size to the pectorals. They also work the hard-to-reach inner pecs, building thick bands of dense muscle throughout their length.

Continuous tension. This is the main rep technique you should use when shape training the chest, or any body part. Continuous tension involves moving through the range of motion as deliberately as possible, almost flexing the muscle throughout the movement. The tighter and slower the movement the better. This type of movement will increase capillary growth and muscle density as well as vascularity.

Continuous tension allows you to use high-intensity training (to momentary muscular failure), with very little risk of injury, especially since isolation exercises and/or machines are utilized in shape training.

Priority exercise selection. When shaping and proportioning the pecs, choose the exercises that directly work the weakest areas first. Each succeeding exercise should be next down the priority list. Work the strongest aspects of the muscle last.

Vince Gironda has written that using only one exercise to stress the slowest growing area of a muscle is the best policy when shape training. This is because the exercise, while stimulating the weak area the most, will also contract the whole muscle and keep the fast growing areas "up." Gironda recommends 10 sets of 10 reps per exercise.

Rep rotation. Each rep comes up through a range of motion slightly differently, which is one reason why free weights are so effective: You never quite do the same motion twice, keeping the muscles and the central nervous system always adapting to new stimuli.

The more diverse the range of motion, the more learning that takes place, and the more adaptations the muscle undergoes. Turning the hands (supinating or pronating, turning outward or inward, respectively) stimulates the proprioceptors in the muscles (sensory end organs in the muscles, tendons and joint capsules), which in turn stimulate the brain's connection with the muscle. This is essentially the same idea as in PNF stretching, except that rotation—not contracting movements—stimulate the adaptation.

Taking the dumbbell or cable flyes purposely through a slightly different path each rep creates exceptional shape in the muscle as it exposes new fibers to the resistance and continually creates new and different hypertrophy adaptations.

You can do your bench presses to the throat one workout, using a medium grip, and the next time take them to the throat, but with a wide grip. You can bring a third of the reps to your throat, a third to the mid-pec line and the last third to the lower-pec line. And you can vary the grip on each of these. The variations are limitless. If you can feel it working where you want to develop the muscle, you are on the right track.

Posing or flexing the muscle against itself is an excellent way, along with stretching exercises, to learn how to recognize what the contracted muscle feels like. Once you know how to contract the muscle in isolation, it will be easier to do under the weights. Trying to "squeeze" the pecs while also trying to survive a heavy bench takes practice and guts. Doing high-rep flexes after you pump the area is an excellent finish to a workout. This is also a place to take advantage of contracting the muscle through as many different lines of pull as possible.

Without total control over where the muscle contractions are placed, the development and shape of the muscle will be haphazard. In the book *Pumping Iron*, authors Charles Gaines and George Butler make note of Ed Corney's intense power of concentration. Sitting in a room packed full of people waiting for the Mr. Universe contest, which Corney was competing in, Corney's concentration was "as apt as any yogi's." He was lost somewhere inside his biceps.

SUPER-, TRI- AND GIANT-SETTING FOR COMPLETE MUSCLE SHAPING

The first one or two exercises you do in a routine receive a disproportionate share of the training energy. If you are focusing on obtaining overall pectoral shape, using straight sets is not the best method. The last exercises in the routine will not get the same intensity as the first. Combining exercises back to back (super-sets), three in a row (tri-sets) or four or more in a row (giant sets) with no rest between them, not only works the muscle intensely but balances the energy that each of the exercises receives.

You will still need to prioritize the order of the exercises, especially in giant sets, but even the last exercise in a giant set will get plenty of stimulation when you are relatively fresh as in the beginning of your workout when priority routines should always be done.

Super-sets work well combining different types of exercises such as Incline Dumbbell Flyes with Incline Dumbbell Presses. Tri-setting can work well with an alternating cycle of exercises so that the weaker triceps don't limit the stimulation the pecs receive. A good shaping tri-set is: Incline Cable Flyes, Flat Bench Dumbbell Press followed by Around-the-World Decline Flyes. This works all areas of the pecs intensely.

For giant sets, pick four or five exercises that work the weakest aspect of your pecs. Let's say your priority is upper pecs. This would be an excellent giant set: Incline Barbell Bench Press, Low Incline Dumbbell Flyes, Dumbbell Pullover, Flat Bench Dumbbell Press, Low Seat Pec Dec Flyes. Do two to three giant sets of 10 to 12 reps each. This routine shapes the upper pecs as well as maintain overall pec mass and shape.

UPPER PEC EMPHASIS

The upper pecs are the hardest area for most bodybuilders to develop and shape. It's important to hit this area from a variety of angles and with relatively high reps. It's also one of the harder areas to keep pumped. One of the best ways to work the upper pecs is with an Incline Fly/Incline Dumbbell Press super-set. By doing the isolation exercise first, you work the pecs directly without help of the triceps. Going immediately to the Incline Dumbbell Presses temporarily makes the triceps stronger than the pecs. This helps create excellent shape as the same area is bombarded with stimulation from the two exercises and a single bench angle.

Do two to three cycles of these two exercises, resting only after each super-set. Do 12 reps per set. Use a different bench angle each set, starting at 20 degrees and increasing one hole each set to 45 degrees.

Next go to Bentover Cable Crossovers, your torso bent at the waist, almost parallel to the floor. Your shoulders should be exactly in line with the two floor pulleys. Draw the handles across the front of your chest to the finished peak contraction position. Let the hands cross at the finished position. Hold the peak contraction for two counts. Do four sets of 15 reps each.

Incline Dumbbell Fly, 4 × 15
Incline Dumbbell Press, 2-3 cycles of 12 reps each
Bentover Cable Crossover, 4 × 15

Cable Flyes can also be performed while standing. Bend your knees slightly to reduce the stress on the lower back.

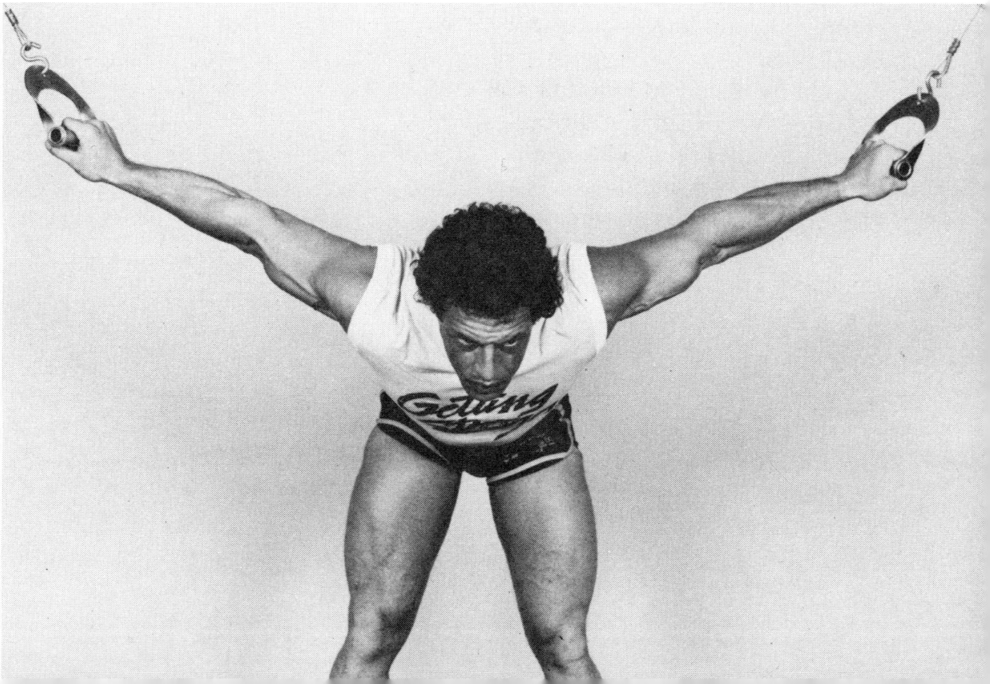

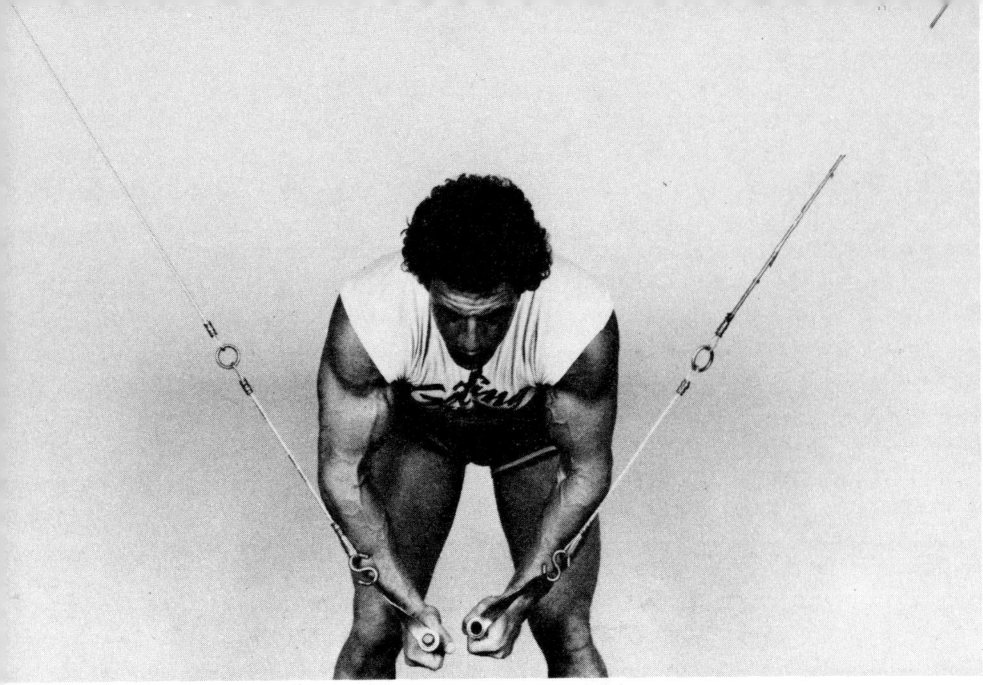

◀ *Your hands should touch lightly at the completion of the Bentover Cable Fly.*

Standing Cable Crossovers work the lower portion of the chest. Start with your hands stretched out as shown. ▼

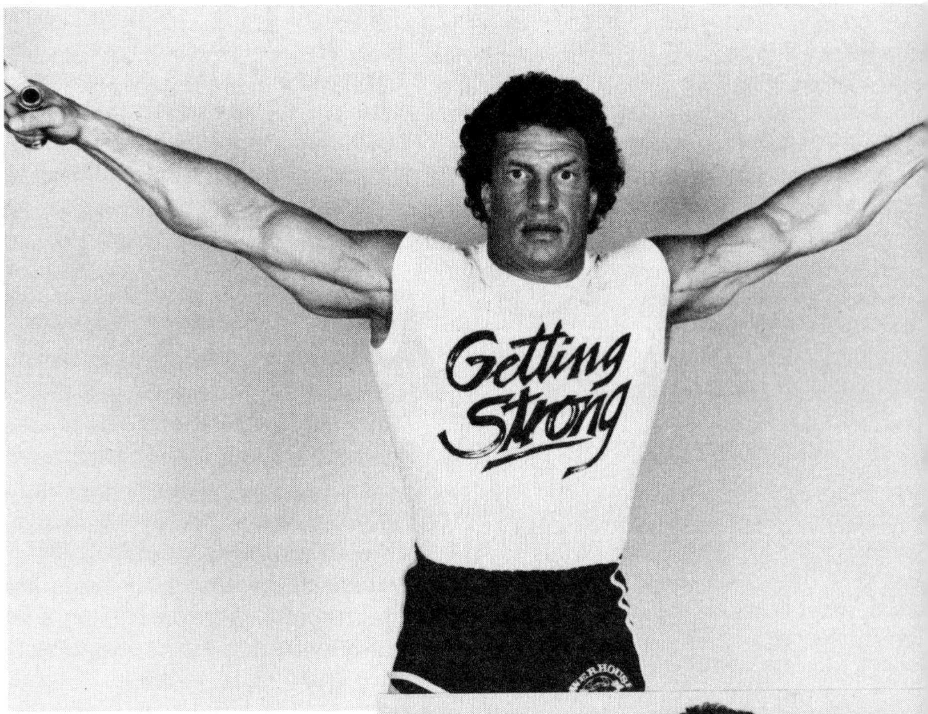

TRI-SETTING FOR CARVED LOWER PECS

Most bodybuilders need to work on their lower pecs. Steve Reeves was noted for his exceptional lower pec development and shape. His pecs had a straight line across the bottom, increasing even more his great width.

Decline Flyes work this area, as do Standing Cable Crossovers when the cable is brought down directly to the sides. Narrow-Grip Dips build and shape the lower pecs, especially the bottom half of the motion.

Begin the tri-set with 45-degree Decline Flyes. With the plates touching, lower the dumbbells in a semicircle behind you until they reach maximum stretch. Sweep the dumbbell up through the same arc, contracting the lower, outer pecs. Do 12 reps.

Go immediately to Standing Cable Crossovers, bringing the cables down directly to the sides and finishing with the handles at your waist. This hits the same area as the Decline Flyes. Do 12 reps. Finish the tri-set with Narrow-Grip Dips, going as low as possible and coming only halfway up. Do as many reps as possible each set.

One tri-set of:	**Reps**
Decline Fly	12 reps
Standing Cable Crossover	12 reps
Narrow-Grip Dip	Max

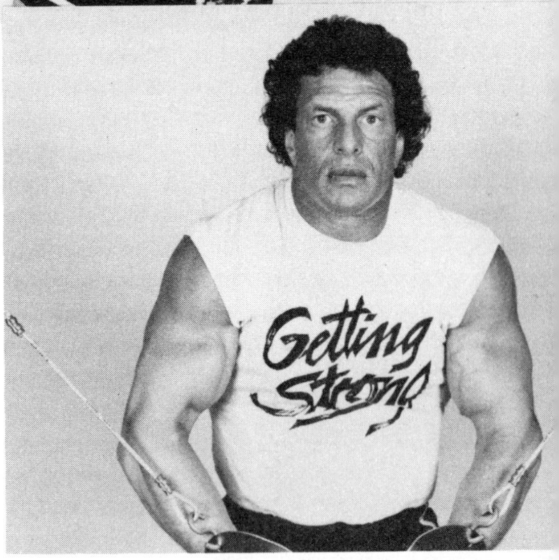

▶ *To fully contract the pecs, bring your hands down and in front of you. Your hands should touch lightly.*

LENGTH CONTRACTION NON-SPECIFIC SHAPING

This routine is excellent after you've been pressing heavy weight for a while. By concentrating solely on length contraction stretching pec exercises, you open and work the pecs in an unusual manner, creating new shape in all parts of the chest.

Start the workout with four sets of 12 reps of the Dumbbell Pullover, cross-bench style to maximize pec stretch. Get your training partner to hold your knees down to further isolate the chest. Tilt the top dumbbell forward on the positive rep to engage the upper pecs.

Go next to Incline Dumbbell Flyes, working the stretch on a 45-degree incline bench. Do four sets of 12. Finish the workout with 45-degree Decline Flyes. You'll confuse the pecs going from a flat stretch, to a high, to a low stretch. If you have a shallow or sunken chest, this routine will work wonders. Do all these pullovers and flyes for high reps and and a sunken chest won't stay sunken for long.

	Sets	Reps
Dumbbell Pullover	4	12
Incline Dumbbell Fly	4	12
Decline Fly	4	12-15

PEAK CONTRACTION THICKNESS ROUTINE

The chest with the nicest shape has thickness and density. When all areas of the chest are large, thick, striated and muscular, the shape of the entire chest is enhanced. Peak contraction exercises such as the primary portion of the Pec Dec, thicken and striate the entire chest. Do Single Cable Crossovers for the inner edge of the pec unilaterally and you can direct intense effort into this very small area.

Peak contraction, continuous tension and intense concentration make this routine effective.

Nautilus Pec Dec—5 sets of 15, 12, 10, 8, 6 reps (add weight each exercise)

Single Arm High Pulley Cable Crossover—2-3 sets of 15 reps

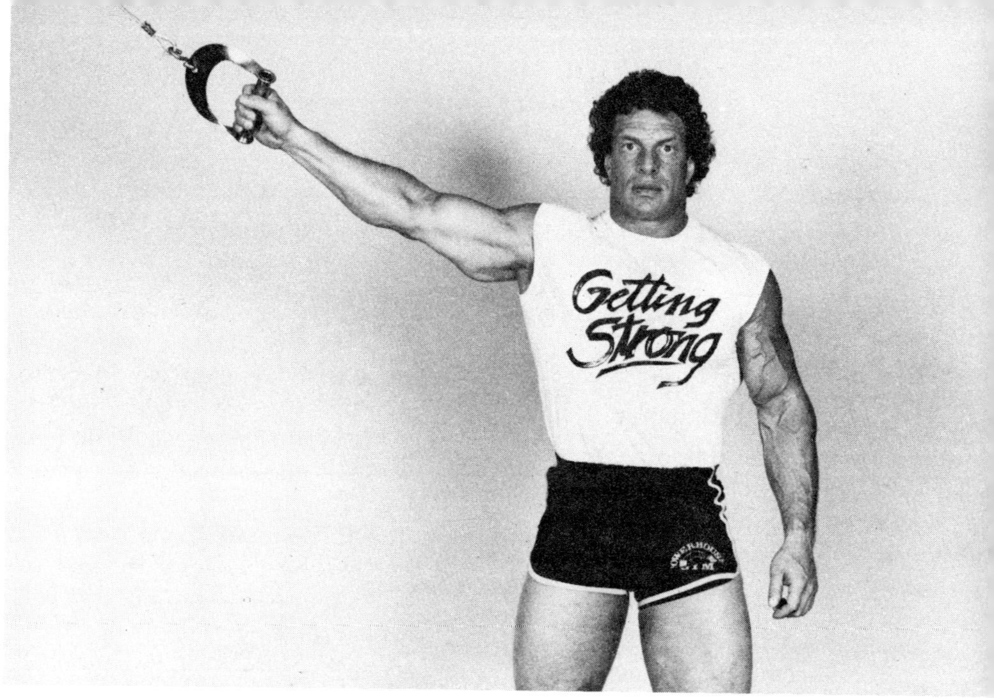

Standing Cable Crossovers can also be performed one arm at a time. Your legs should be shoulder-width apart or slightly wider for balance.

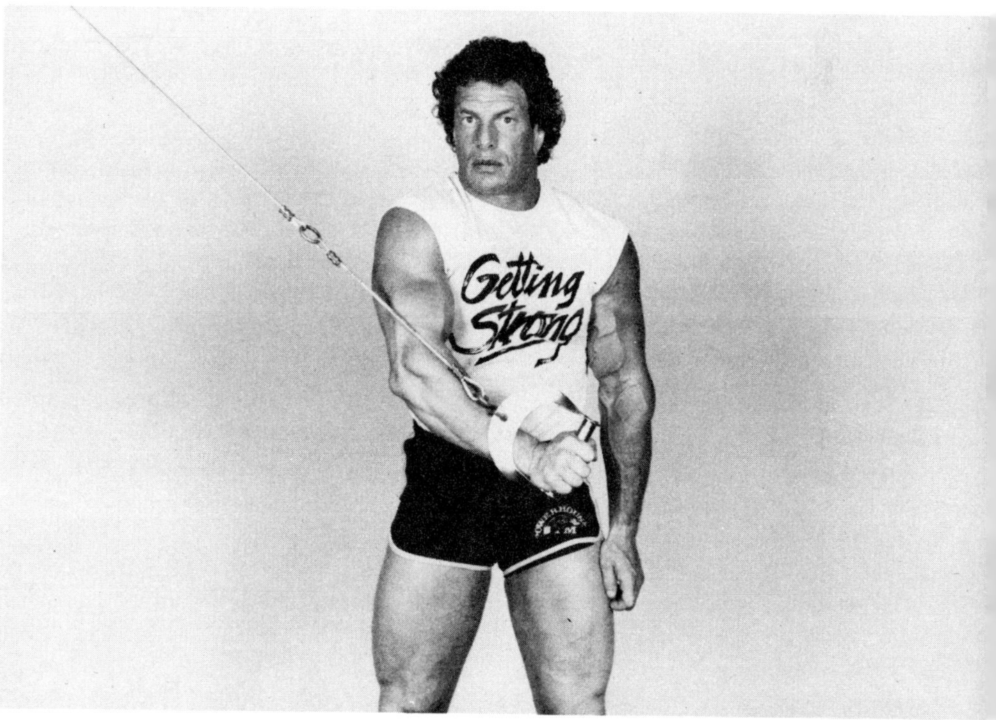

Professional bodybuilder Don Ross demonstrates proper form on the Single Arm High Pulley Cable Crossover. You must bring your hands down and in front of you for proper emphasis on your pecs.

ISOLATION COMPOUND EXERCISE SHAPE ROUTINE

The easiest way to shape the pecs with barbell compound exercises is using a wide grip and by bringing the bar back to the throat during the Bench Press. This position doesn't stretch the pecs as well as a closer grip, but it effectively isolates the shoulders and triceps out of the exercise and stresses mainly the pecs. Mohammed Makkawy, who has some of the most incredibly carved and visually informative pecs around, uses these often. Do five sets of 10 reps.

Thirty-two inch Parallel Bar Dips work the area right under the armpit, the mid-outer edge of the pecs. This is one of the important "outer" sections that Vince Gironda is always talking about developing to create the greatest width possible. It works, too. Using body weight only, do sets of 12 to 15, working for a burn and pump with as little rest between sets as possible. Do four sets of as many reps as possible.

Low Incline Dumbbell Presses with the palms parallel the entire set isolate the upper pecs well, the hand position keeping the shoulders and pecs out of the action as much as possible. Keep the elbows back as much as possible and lower the dumbbells as if they were a solid bar and you were lowering it to your throat; keep the palms facing each other. Do four set of eight.

	Sets	Reps
Flat Bench Barbell Press to Throat	5	10
Wide Bar Dip	4	max
Low Incline Dumbbell Press (palms parallel)	4	8

SINGLE EXERCISE PRIORITY SHAPING ROUTINES

Let your present pec weakness determine how you choose the exercises in this routine. A very good pectoral shape plan would be to prioritize your chest weak points and plan an all-out assault: do four weeks of one exercise, four weeks of another and four more weeks of a third. Then start the cycle over. By the time you get back to the first exercise, the specific muscle area will be ready for a new growth cycle.

Upper Pecs: Incline Dumbbell Press, Barbell Incline Press (wide or shoulder-width grip), Dumbbell Pullover, Upright Cable Fly, Bent Cable Crossover, Low Seat Pec Dec, Incline Dumbbell Fly.

Lower Pecs: Decline Fly, Decline Press (barbell or dumbbell), Narrow-Grip Parallel Bar Dip, Standing Cable Crossover, Polaris "Crusher" Pec Dec, Nautilus Decline Press, Power Bench Press (to sternum), Decline Cable Fly, Flat Bench Dumbbell Press, Around-the-World Fly

Inner Pecs: Any peak contraction Pec Dec, Peak Contraction Cable Crossover (uni- or bilateral), Narrow-Grip Bench Press

Outer Pecs: Flat Bench Fly, Flat Bench Wide-Grip Bench Press, Flat Bench Cable Fly, Wide Bar Parallel Bar Dip

Mid Pecs: Shoulder-Width Bench Press (barbell), Round Back Dip (narrow bars) Flat Bench Dumbbell Press (palms turned away), Dumbbell Pullover (cross bench)

POSING FOR MUSCLE SHAPE

Regardless of whether you want to be a competitive bodybuilder or not, learning to pose the muscle will enhance the muscle's shape and your ability to mentally connect with the muscle.

Pose or tense the muscle as often as possible. If you do not feel comfortable posing in the gym between sets, go to the locker room and tense those pecs where you can be alone. Try to "bring out" the details that you want to appear. Try to "find" them, feeling them contract as deeply as possible.

It's preferable to pose the muscle when it is pumped up, between sets or body parts, as this gives you even better muscle control. However, it is extremely difficult to get a pumped up, fatigued muscle to contract. Solve this problem by doing repetition flexes through the pose's range of motion. Do the pose, hold for a tight contraction, release and repeat as many times as necessary to fatigue the pecs.

TEN: DEFINITION TRAINING

Proper bodybuilding training builds muscle mass. If that muscle mass is hidden under a layer of fat, you can have all the lines, separation and definition in the world on your pecs and no one will ever see them.

Most people who train with weights for a period of time build more muscle. And yet the overall look is usually not one of definition and muscularity but of "bulk." Even at less body weight you will look bigger and more impressive if you concentrate on gaining quality muscle mass and staying that way.

Let's look at definition. A defined muscle is one that stands out from the rest. The upper, lower, inner and outer sections of the muscle are plainly visible. You can tell where the shoulder stops and the pecs begin. Definition used to be simple. The muscle group had to be separated from the rest.

Today it is not enough, for the competitive bodybuilder at least, to be just defined. He or she must have good upper and lower pectoral separation, clearly carved lower pecs separated from the abs, serratus muscles, sternal development and separation that looks like little fingers on the inner pecs. He or she needs a total complement of striations across the entire pecs, and vascularity, emphasizing the low levels of body fat. That is the modern version of definition, but now it's called the ripped or the shredded look.

Some people say today's bodybuilders are too defined. But the look is winning and more and more people want to know how to define and "rip" their own physiques.

The most obvious hindrance to good pec definition is subcutaneous body fat. The trick is to lose the body fat covering your precious pecs without losing the muscle mass that makes them so precious. You must keep the intensity of the workouts high, focusing on contracting the pecs to their fullest to create separation, striations and muscularity.

The key to losing body fat is the calorie. Take in more than your daily maintenance level, and on comes the adipose tissue. Most assume the best way to lose body fat is to eat less. This usually works in reverse. If you continually drop calories from the diet, the body thinks you are starving it and it starts to counteract your definition efforts!

The first thing it does is lower your metabolism. You feel more sluggish, want to do less and feel like burning fewer calories. A starving body thinks this is just grand.

The next thing the body does is start to store fat. Yes, you read right. Fat has the most calories pound for pound, so a starving body will go for fat as the fuel of choice.

The best way to lose weight is not just dieting, but cutting calories and increasing aerobic activity at the same time. Most bodybuilders think that the only place to get an aerobic effect is in the exercise cycle or by running. But quality training also works—reducing rest levels between exercises progressively, super-, tri- and giant setting. You can increase the workload on the muscle while increasing calories burned, and you can create an aerobic effect from the lack of rest periods between sets.

Working an isolated muscle aerobically will maximize the endurance systems in the muscle. Although the body loses fat all over, burning the intramuscular fat from a heavily used muscle will create a leaner muscle.

Just think, if spot reducing is totally bunk, then why do you see marathoners with incredibly defined legs and "love handles" around the middle, an area almost unused in the running motion?

The best way to create definition in the pectorals is a combination of lowering your caloric intake while creating a calorie deficiency through general aerobic (walking, running) training and specific aerobic training for the chest. You must remember, though, to keep your strength up in at least one basic exercise.

Going hand-in-hand with proper aerobic training is the importance of proper food selection and supplements for the diet. When you are trying to get your body fat down with extra training while on a reduced calorie diet, your intake of vital nutrients will suffer. Supplements keep any deficiencies from occurring.

When you are definition training, you are trying to get your body to burn "hot." If you have all the proper nutrients available, the body can rev up to what is required. If it has do go searching for the right tools for the job, it obviously is not going to burn fat as efficiently.

The best definition foods are those low in fat and high in lean protein or complex carbohydrates. The easiest way to drop calories without being hungry is the low-fat, high carbohydrate diet.

Higher Reps

Top bodybuilders usually use higher rep schemes while training for definition and muscularity. This is done to: 1) enhance the mind/body connection for better hardness and striations, 2) work the mitochondria and capillary systems, 3) create density and muscularity, 4) burn intramuscular fat and 5) create a faster metabolism.

Exercise Combinations

In order to maximize muscle shape and definition, super-sets, tri-sets and giant sets are frequently used. Combine the priority shaping exercises discussed earlier.

Isolation Exercises/Higher Sets

Isolation exercises will give the best results. You must maintain muscle mass with occasional strength training, but most of your energy should be directed to unilateral (one arm) and bi-lateral isolation exercises. This maximizes neurological benefit in a muscle area, creating the striations and lines that you see as definition.

Doing more reps with less weight inflicts less stress to the system than does high-intensity, low-rep sets: You can do more sets with less strain, burn more calories, do more work to etch in detail and expose the muscle to more exercise angles.

You can also work the muscle more frequently when training for definition. The muscles recover from high-rep training stress faster than absolute high-intensity training. High intensity training, remember, refers to using as complete an effort as possible during an exercise. You can go to failure with One-Arm Cable Crossovers and it will be intense, but not at the same level of intensity as going to failure with very heavy power bench presses.

Sunbathing

Yes sunbathing! Progressive and regular sunbathing can increase the definition of your entire body. The sun seems to melt the fat off the muscles, but what's really happening is that the water underneath the skin is lost, temporarily creating better separation and tone. By keeping your salt intake down and increasing natural sources of potassium (fresh fruit, veggies) you can "relocate" the water from outside the muscle cell to inside the cell, where it makes the muscle look bigger and improves definition.

When you sweat, sodium is lost from the body with the water. Most people take in 10 to 20 times the amount of sodium necessary for a healthy diet (500-1000 mg.). The bronze look you get from sunbathing and a diet high in potassium and low in sodium can increase your definition 100 percent.

CHEST DEFINITION ROUTINES

Since you can work all the areas of the chest and save energy by doing giant sets, use this technique frequently for definition training. By using isolation or compound exercises you will be able to work deeper into the muscle, creating more lines and separation with the multiangle technique.

Always try to set up the equipment you will be needing in advance so you will waste no time getting from exercise to exercise, the essential component in giant setting. Rest as little as possible during the giant set, but take as much rest as necessary between giant sets.

Multiangular Isolation Giant Sets

Here's the repetition scheme on each of the three cycles you will do. On the first cycle, use Standing Cable Crossovers to hit the general pec area with a set of 10 reps, as heavy as possible. Go immediately to the Pec Dec. Use continuous tension and peak contractions for another set of 10. Stretch the pecs next with Cross Bench Dumbbell Pullovers for 10 reps. Finish the giant set with Decline Flyes on a 45-degree decline for a blistering set of 10 reps.

Do the same exercises in the same sequence for the second cycle but use 12 reps per set. Fire out 15 reps on each exercise for the third and last cycle. The pecs will pump on this progressive reps system. The next workout, do the same exercises but in a different sequence.

THREE-CYCLE GIANT SETS

Standing Cable Crossover 1×10, 12, 15 reps

Nautilus Pec Dec 1×10, 12, 15 reps

Cross Bench Dumbbell Pullover 1×10, 12, 15 reps

Decline Fly 1×10, 12, 15 reps

Compound Exercise Giant Set for Calorie Burn-Off

Although isolation exercises are superb for building shape and striations into the pecs, they do not work as many muscles as compound exercises, so they do not burn as many calories. Weight training is not a good method of burning calories, but the more muscles involved in each exercise the more calories burned.

Begin the giant set with Medium-Grip Bench Presses on a flat bench. Work for upper pec isolation, bringing the bar to your throat. Do 10 reps. Go next to Wide-Grip Gironda Dips keeping the chin on the chest and focusing on the lower, outer pecs. Go back to the upper pecs with 45-degree Incline Dumbbell Presses with the palms facing away the entire set. Shock the pecs now by going to the lower pecs with Decline Barbell Bench Presses. Do 10 reps for each exercise.

This routine will effectively blast the triceps, so don't worry too much about the weights used. When you get to the last two exercises, your pressing muscles will be pretty tired. This is what makes the routine so effective, though, so use weights that you can control and force out those reps. The pecs will be aching by the second giant set, but do three cycles.

	Sets	Reps
Medium-Grip Barbell Bench Press	1	10
Wide-Grip Gironda Dip	1	10
Incline Dumbbell Press	1	10
Decline Barbell Press	1	10

Alternating Pre-Exhaust Giant Set

By working in pre-exhaust fashion from the upper to lower pecs, you create stress deep in the muscle from top to bottom and from side to side.

Have all the benches set up so you can move from exercise to exercise as quickly as possible. Start with Low Incline Dumbbell Flyes, doing 10 reps each, and go immediately into Dumbbell Presses, palms facing each other for 10 reps. Move from the incline bench to a prone position on the flat bench for Dumbbell Flyes, followed by Flat Bench Dumbbell Presses with the palms facing away from the body. Use 10 reps on each exercise.

Go quickly to the decline bench and pump out 10 reps of Decline Flyes with as much weight as your pecs can handle. Finish with Decline Dumbbell Presses. Start the press with the palms facing away and turn them in as the dumbbells descend. Turn the dumbbells away from your palms as you press back up.

	Sets	Reps
Incline Dumbbell Fly	1	10
Incline Dumbbell Press (palms parallel)	1	10
Flat Bench Dumbbell Fly	1	10
Flat Bench Dumbbell Press (palms forward)	1	10
Decline Dumbbell Fly	1	10
Decline Dumbbell Press (rotating hands)	1	10

Go through two cycles on each exercise.

Double Pre-Exhaust Tri-Set

By going from an isolation exercise to a compound exercise, the pecs are continually stressed. When the triceps give out in the compound exercise, the pecs might still have some unstimulated muscle fibers. By going right back after them with a lighter isolation exercise that continues to stimulate muscle, every fiber will be worked. That is a double pre-exhaust tri-set.

Start the exercise with High Incline (60-degree) Dumbbell Flyes, reaching out to the sides as much as possible. This works the clavicle area of the upper pecs. Go next to Wide-Grip Gironda Flyes, trying for as many reps as possible. When a full rep is no longer possible, lower into the full stretch position and do bottom-half push outs, for the lower pec fibers. Come from the full stretch to halfway up and then lower and repeat.

After the pecs are tired from dips, go back to flyes, this time doing Steep Decline Dumbbell Flyes (50 to 60 degrees for 12 reps) to complete one cycle. Do three to four tri-sets for maximum definition stimulation.

Remember, light weights are only good for stopping doors. Learn to think in terms of heavy low reps, heavy medium reps and heavy high reps. If the work isn't enough to overload, you will fail to develop.

Routines for definition or for any type of adaptation that are not progressive are maintenance routines. Your body will change shape or strengthen only when it is asked to do a task that requires increased muscle adaptation.

Progressive Rep Push-Ups

This is an excellent workout should you need to train without equipment. Start by doing a set of Medium-Grip Push-ups (or push-ups between chairs), touching your chest to the floor. Count the reps. Take as much rest as necessary to regain your breath and try for the same amount of reps plus two more.

The third set should include two extra reps also. For the fourth set, decrease the reps by four, working for a stricter motion. The fifth and sixth sets should reduce the reps by four each time, the movement getting slower and stricter with each set; work for as much pec isolation as possible.

By the end of this routine your pecs should be pumped to the max. This is also an excellent method for training the chest muscle for endurance.

Multiangle High-Rep Push-Up Routine

The major drawbacks to push-ups are: lack of a stretch, the inability to increase the resistance and the limited number of angles to use. Push-up routines are best saved for emergencies so the stress will be as unfamiliar as possible for better adaptation.

This routine works around some of the problems by having you do push-ups from different angles, and creating a stretch for the pecs at the same time.

Start the push-up routine with Upper Chest Push-ups, your hands shoulder-width apart on the floor and your feet propped up on a stool or bench. Do 20 reps. Go next to push-ups between two chairs with both feet on a third chair behind you. Keep the chairs wide to work the outer pecs and stretch as deeply as possible. Do 20 reps. Finish the tri-set with regular floor push-ups, elbows out to the sides and hands turned in; do 20 reps. Do three to four of these tri-sets.

Cable Definition Routine

Cables provide continuous tension on the pecs to help bring out definition. The muscle fibers are exposed to stress throughout the range of motion.

Start with Standing Cable Crossovers. Stand straight with arms overhead and out to the sides and bring each cable handle down, finishing with the handles in front of the waist. Hold each rep for two seconds at the finish position. Do four sets of 12 reps each.

Next go to Bentover Cable Crossover with the same pulley crossover machine. Bend forward and keep the shoulders in line with the pulleys as you bring the arms together in front of your chest. Do four sets of 12.

Finish the cable routine with Incline Cable Flyes, working the incline from 60 degrees down to 40; lower the bench after each set. Work the flyes from a full stretch to peak contraction.

	Sets	Reps
Standing Cable Crossover	4	12
Bentover Cable Crossover	4	12
Varying Incline Cable Fly	4	12

By placing your feet on a bench, you can make the push-up emphasize the upper pecs.

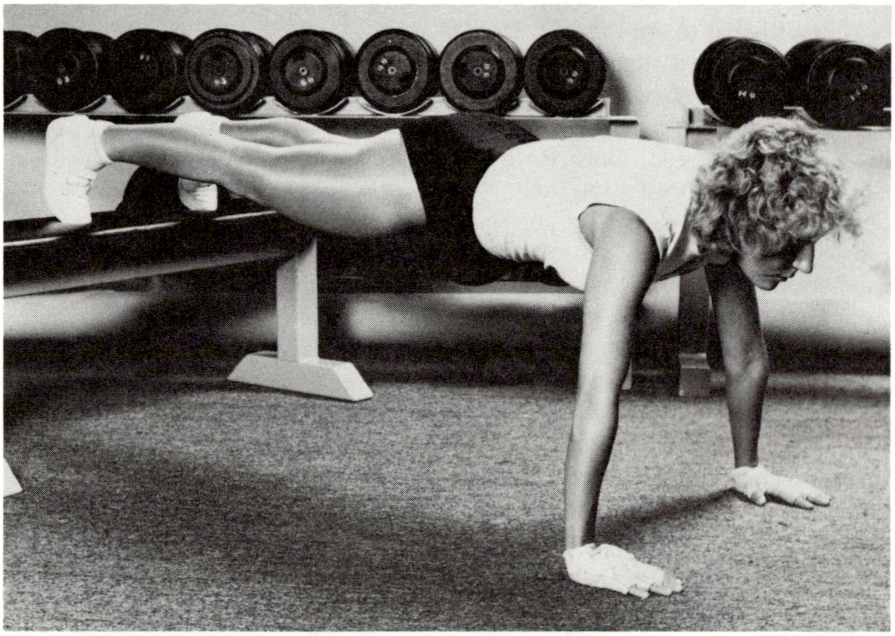

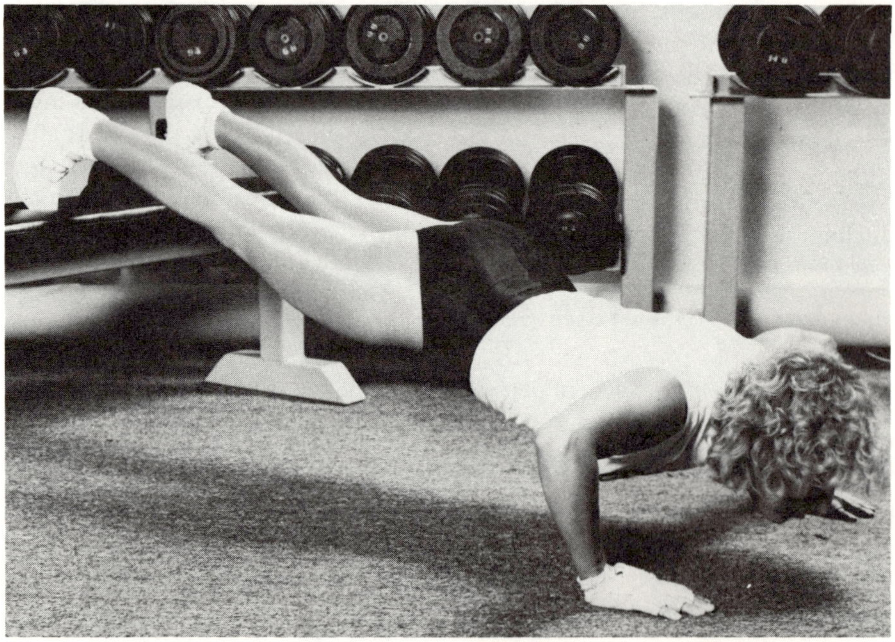

To get a full stretch, keep your elbows out to your sides as you descend into the bottom position of the push-up.

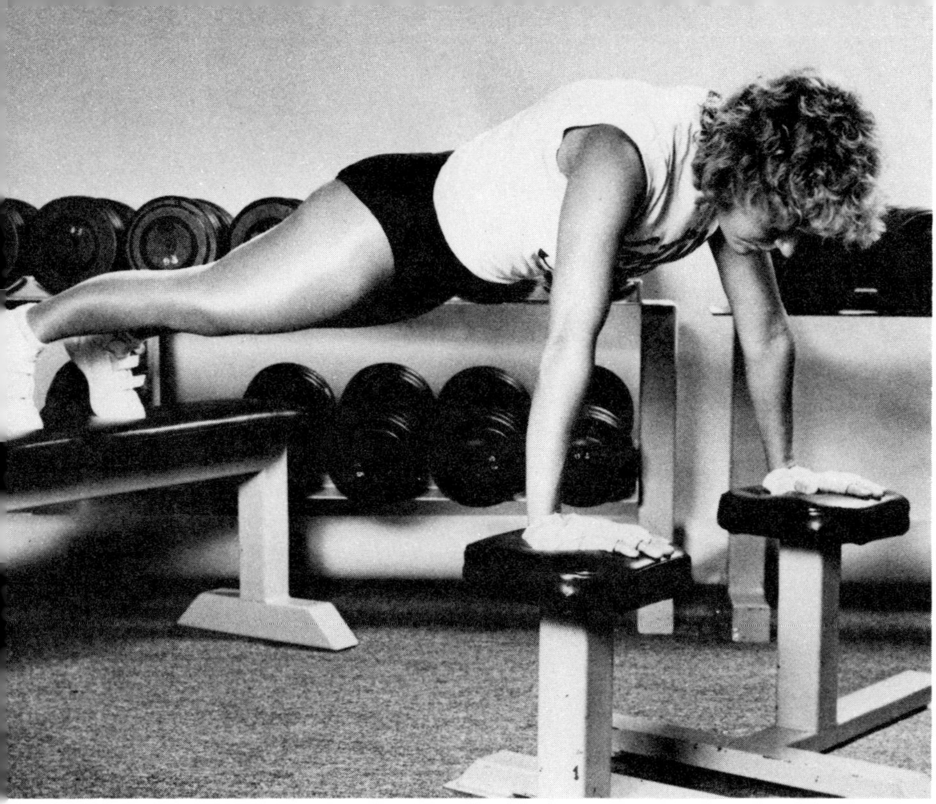

This is the starting position of the Push-up Between Benches. This variation increases the stretch on the pecs.

333'S The Burner

Nothing makes the pecs burn like this series of half and full reps on the simple barbell Bench Press. But nothing forces the pecs to work harder, either. This is an excellent routine for when you are short on time in the gym or you want to isolate the middle part of the pecs.

Start the exercise by doing 11 half reps from the bottom of the bench press to mid-way up. After 11 half reps from the bottom, do 11 half reps from lockout position to mid-way down. This is a little easier and lulls you into a false sense of security, setting you up for the most productive part of the set: Do 11 full reps!

Getting through even one series of these is hard, so for outrageously defined pecs do three! Use a medium to wide grip on the bar and have a training partner hold his hand at the point you need to bring the bar and help you count your reps. Always have a spotter on this one.

Barbell Bench Press From Chest to Halfway Up—11 reps
Barbell Bench Press From Top of Rep to Halfway Down—11 reps
Barbell Bench Press, full reps—11 reps

Pec Dec Tri-Setting Specialization

The inner sections of the pecs are stimulated from this exercise better than any other, and the Pec Dec is probably more responsible for the quality of pecs today at physique shows than any other exercise.

You should take advantage of the various brands of Pec Decs and their slightly different lines of pull. Ideally, you should start the tri-set with the Nautilus Pec Dec, setting the seat low to hit the upper pecs. Do a slow continuous 10 reps. Go immediately to a Polaris Pec Dec with the seat set so that the mid-pecs get stressed the most. Do 10 slow hard reps. Finish the tri-set with the Polaris "Crusher" Pec Dec, which will carve and define the lower/inner pecs. Do 10 reps. Do three to four tri-sets.

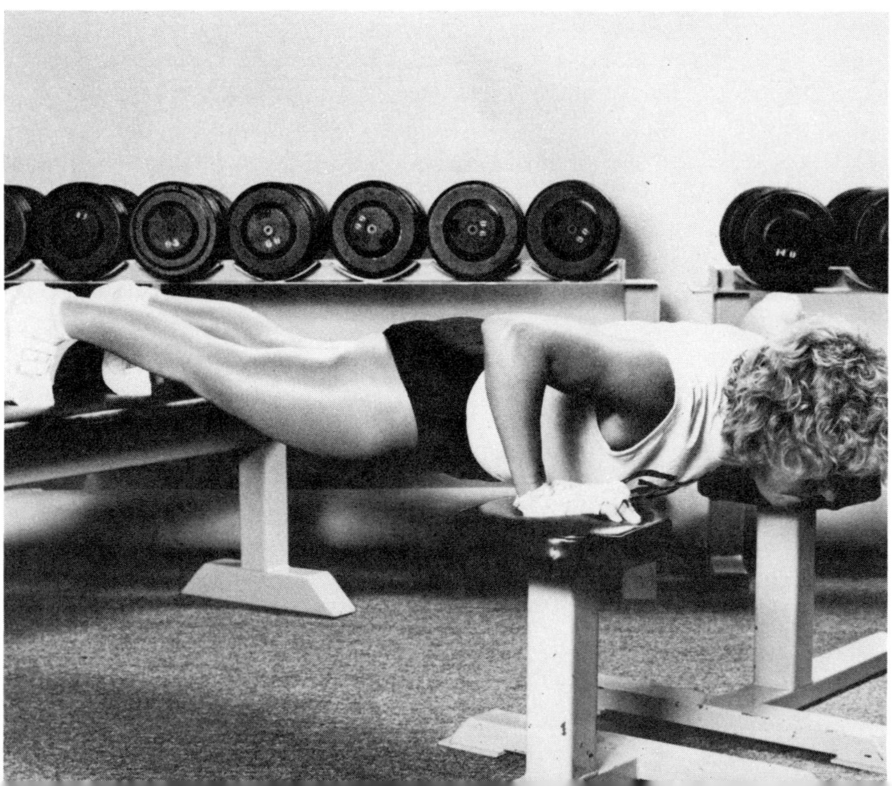

As with the standard push-up, your elbows should point out to your sides during the Push-up Between Benches.

ELEVEN: STRENGTH TRAINING

The Barbell Bench Press is one of the most popular movements ever done with weights! If you have a large muscular-looking chest, the first question asked by many bodybuilders will be: "How much can you bench?"

For strength training the chest, nothing can beat the Barbell Bench Press. Not only does training the chest for strength give you confidence and power, but using the Barbell and Dumbbell Bench Presses as the center of your training is going to give you a big upper body as well!

These lifts, when done with a power style, work every muscle in your upper body. After a hard day of power benches, my pecs are fried, but so are my lats, delts and triceps. Tightening the upper body with vice-like strength, holding the shoulder blades together and keeping the shoulders flat on the bench exposes the entire body to the heaviest overload possible.

Powerlifters, through years of training for the perfect bench groove, lift incredible amounts of weights even in the lighter weight classes. Rick Weil of Suncoast Gym has done 501 pounds in the gym and almost as much in competition at a body weight of only 165 pounds. Muscle size and strength are related only to a point. After that, good leverage (arm/torso proportions, and so on), technique, cell density and neurological ability (the ability to contract muscle fibers) matter more than size, although fat cells, on lifters in heavy classes, can provide some extra leverage, as would a thicker and bigger muscle cell.

The powerlifting mentality is one of success and faith. Powerlifters believe they have no limits. This is true because the heroic act of finding the edge of your strength and power pushes you to your limits. Pushing to the limit is what allows a powerlifter to get stronger into his forties and fifties!

I like to combine the powerlifting mentality with a bodybuilder's concentration and contraction control. I call this power bodybuilding. The foundation of the natural physique and the result of strength training the chest is a density and thickness that immediately identifies you as a strong and powerful person.

STRENGTH TRAINING PRINCIPLES

Strength training is very easy to understand. The basis is lifting very heavy weights for low reps with very good form. Perfect form is essential because the greater the load you are working with, the less margin for error. Make a mistake with a 300-pound bench press and the damage won't be that great. Make the same mistake with 400 pounds and the damage can take months to recover from, keeping you out of training and from making progress.

The better your technique, the better your strength will be. As I noted earlier, the reason you make so much progress as a beginner is because your body is rapidly learning the technique of the lift. The more efficient your central nervous system becomes with a technique, the fewer unnecessary movements and wasted energy you'll suffer from.

You must train heavy with any repetition scheme you are employing if you want to make progress. The muscle only adapts if exposed to an overload. To get a strength adaptation, you must train with a workload in the range of 85 to 95 percent of your max for low reps.

Doing low reps is a confusing term because it means different things to different athletes. Bodybuilders who are strength training should do from four to eight reps as their low-rep range. Powerlifters can also benefit from reps in that range, but to become proficient in lifting a very heavy weight for one rep, you must practice that skill. So lifts would be in the order of 90 to 95 percent of maximum for one to three reps.

Dr. Fred Hatfield (Dr. Squat), an editor of *Muscle and Fitness* magazine and world champion (1983) in the 220-pound class, believes single reps should not be done in practice. He thinks that by using higher reps the body is better conditioned for the heavy single rep. Doing single reps in practice, he believes, only exposes the athlete to unnecessary injuries. Training is for building strength, he believes, and that is best accomplished with three to five sets of four to eight reps.

Multijoint compound exercises are best because they work the involved muscles more intensely, and the body as a whole. By working with exercises that strengthen the body as a whole, explosive and powerful strength can be obtained. Isolation exercises should be secondary, mainly used to strengthen the joint stabilizers, which helps prevent injury.

Training for chest strength requires you to guard against injuring the shoulders and the elbows by also doing sets of higher reps (12 to 15) to promote circulation, connective tissue strength and capillarization, all important in preventing joint injury. Focus on a controlled, full range of motion, peak contraction and continuous tension.

Explosive Power

You should practice explosive power training if you wish to be as strong as possible. Explosive training recruits the most white, fast-twitch fibers. These are the ones primarily responsible for improving strength and size. But realize that when you are training with your heaviest weights (80 to 90 percent of maximum), you cannot lift the weight fast. The load is too heavy for the bar to travel fast. The lift is done explosively, but the bar moves slowly.

Training for that explosiveness is best done with lighter loads so that you can practice being explosive—moving mass at speed. The Russians do different types of movements for explosive training for strength, such as broad and vertical jumping, long jumping for repetitions, shock jumping, or jumping off a small table into a deep squat and rebounding as fast as possible.

The reason for all this jumping is because it teaches explosiveness, a learned trait. It teaches the body to recruit muscle fiber faster, which gives you greater power and allows you to lift more weight.

Recovery: The Essential Ingredient

Training is only half the equation. The other, almost more important half, is recovery from a particular training load. Overload strength training is designed to ask from your body a little more than it has given before. After the body has rested and reabsorbed all the nutrients it needs, it will adapt to this new stress with the adaptation that the load stimulated, either strength or endurance or a combination of many stimuli.

Training with high-intensity loads every day will prevent recovery and eventually preclude high-intensity training itself! You must give your body time to do its job and recover from breakdown. The stronger you get, the more the stress. Among the strongest people in the world, powerlifters, training the bench press heavy only once a week is popular. Why? Because when 90 percent of your max is still over 400 pounds, you are undergoing extensive tissue breakdown. An equally extensive recovery period is needed.

The upper body muscles recover faster than the legs, though, so they can handle more training sessions per week. But I still recommend only benching heavy once a week. By the time you get back to the Bench Press, you should be recovered enough to use maximal weights and achieve the necessary overload.

Training the bench heavy only once a week is also easier on you mentally. Getting up for a hard workout with heavy weights is much easier if you have recovered physically and mentally from the last session. Many lifters, though, like to include a lighter bench day to work on technique, explosiveness or bodybuilding. I've had the best strength results from training the chest once a week as heavy as possible on an inverted pyramid—15, 12, 10, 8 and 6 reps—with Incline Flyes and Cable Crosses for assistance chest work.

When you know you only have one shot a week to get in a great workout, there is a tendency to take it more seriously and work harder. If you mess up, you have to wait another week to pump your chest. But if you do it right, you shouldn't need to train your chest again for a week.

STRENGTH TRAINING ROUTINES

Basic Power

This is the most basic power chest routine you can do. There are no frills, just hard work. In strength training, even more so than with shape, definition or size training, quantity will never substitute for quality. To maximize each set, form and technique should be understood and practiced as perfectly as possible, both in physical and mental training. Practice, a good gymnastics friend of mine always says, does not make perfect, it makes permanent. If you practice bad form, that's what you will get: perfectly bad form.

Do this routine once a week on

the same days as shoulders and arms.

Start with the power Bench Press, working four sets of 10, 8, 6, and then one very heavy set of six. If you need help on any of these sets, this should be the one. Be conservative on the first three, but use a heavy weight. You should be able to make all the reps yourself. On the last set, pick a weight you know you can get four or five from, and then push yourself to six. Do it all on your own.

Go next to a Narrow-Grip Bench Press with a straight bar, hands one inch apart. Lower your elbows directly to your sides and explode from the bottom. Do four sets of five reps, as heavy as possible. Increase the weight when you can get all four sets of five.

Next go to Parallel Dips to finish the pushing muscles with a great pump. Keep a power dip position, going down for chest isolation (feet in front, chin down) and powering up through the triceps. Do four sets of as many reps as possible each set. Get a deep stretch each set.
Hammer Curls (alternate Dumbbell Curls done with the hands parallel, thumbs up the entire set) work the muscles of the forearms and biceps, building, in essence, a launching pad for the bottom of the Bench Press. Biceps are used extensively when lowering the bar on the Bench Press, help keep the elbow joint strong and help launch those heavy benches for better chest development and strength. Do four sets of eight.

	Sets	Reps
Barbell Power Bench Press	4	10, 8 6, 6
Narrow-Grip Bench Press	4	5
Body Weight Dip	4	max
Dumbbell Hammer Curl	4	8

DUMBBELL POWER BENCH TRAINING

Dumbbells have these advantages over the barbell: provide a greater range of motion, work each side of the body more completely, are harder to use because they require more coordination and joint strength, and can be done alone safely. Given all these advantages, heavy dumbbell training should be a regular part of your chest work.

The bigger and stronger your chest gets, the less benefit you will receive from barbell training, owing to a decreasing range of motion. Including heavy dumbbell benches and incline benches will keep the strength of your range of motion deep. This is also essential for strong connective tissue and joint integrity.

Another reason for doing heavy dumbbell pressing is because it's fun. There's something primal and animalistic about carrying around huge, ominous dumbbells. Imagine yourself holding one of the Norse god's, Thor, mighty hammers in each hand! Dumbbell pressing also allows you the luxury of training with very heavy weights by yourself. If you try this with barbells, there is always the danger of becoming pinned during a workout. This does happen, so no one should train heavy benches without a spotter. It's too dangerous and too easy to make a mistake.

But with heavy dumbbells, even if you miss the rep completely, you can always get out from under them safely. For those without regular training partners, heavy dumbbell training is the way to go.

Dumbbell Press

Start the workout with flat bench Dumbbell Presses, turning the palms in as you lower the weights and turning palms out as you raise them. After a light warmup do max sets of 15, 12, 10, 8 and 6 reps. Go for the heaviest weight possible on that last set of six.

Incline Dumbbell Press

Go next to Incline Dumbbell Presses with the same hand rotations, palms in as you lower the

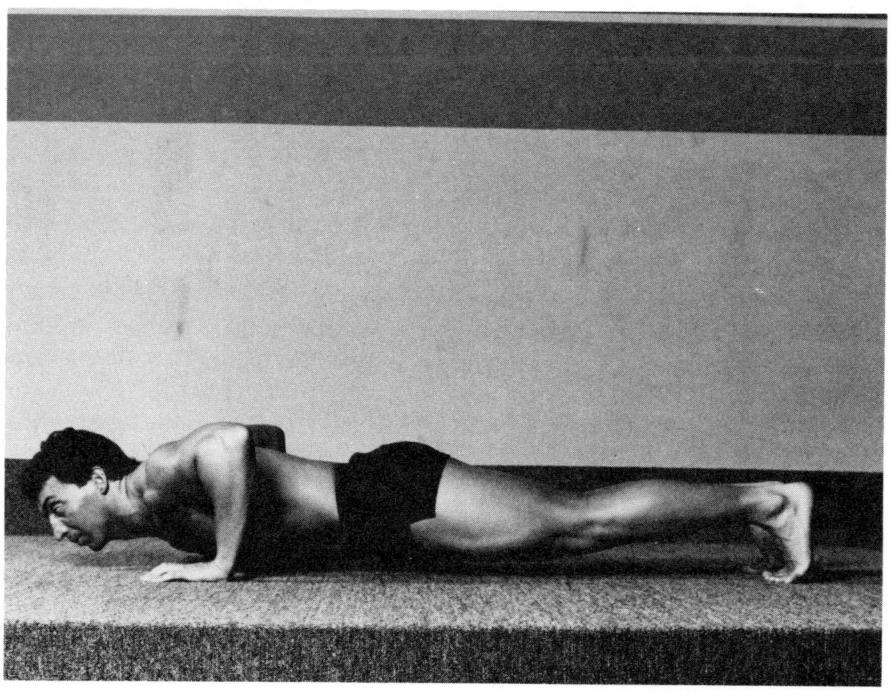

This is one of the classic speed training exercises for the chest. Begin as in a standard push-up, but blast yourself into an airborne position, using explosive arm power for maximum muscular stimulation.

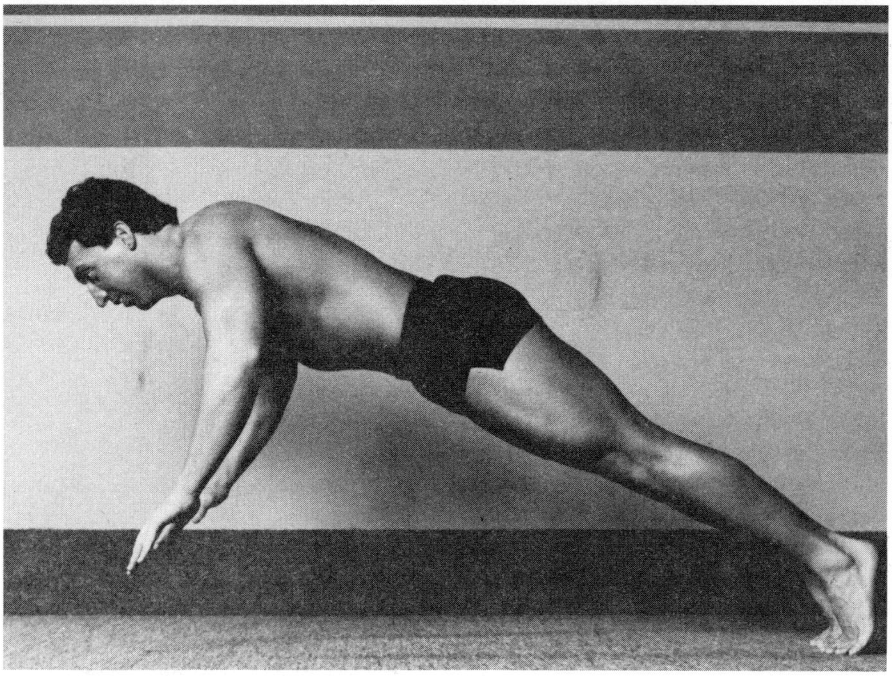

As you blast yourself away from the floor, be sure to maintain proper form.

weight, palms out as you raise it. Use a fairly steep (50 to 70 degree) incline bench for these. Again, do 15, 12, 10, 8 and 6 reps, each set as heavy as possible.

Explosion Push-up

Next, go to Explosion Push-ups, lowering slowly between two chairs (feet up on a third) and do the positive rep as powerfully as possible. Be very careful with this type of training! Never lose form, especially after the push out from the bottom. You should focus on attaining the perfect stretch, pause in that stretch and then speed out of the bottom, striving for as integrated an effort from the pecs, delts and triceps as possible. Do three sets of 10 to 12 reps.

Lat Machine Pushdown, Alternate Front Raise and Side Laterals

Finish the routine with Lat Machine Pressdowns for the triceps, and Alternate Front Raises and Side Laterals for shoulder stability. Do three sets of 10 for each exercise. Do this routine once a week with shoulders and arms.

Flat Bench Dumbbell Press—5 sets of 15, 12, 10, 8, 6
Incline Dumbbell Press—5 sets of 15, 12, 10, 8, 6
Explosion Push-up—3 sets 10-12
Triceps Pressdown—3 × 10
Lat Machine Pushdown—3 × 10
Alternate Front Raise—3 × 10
Side Lateral—3 × 10

THE SUPER STRETCH BENCH PRESS ROUTINE

As with the dumbbell routine just mentioned, this routine emphasizes stretching the chest. The stronger you are in the first portion of the bench press, the easier the lift will be. It will be like having to do only a half a rep when you are used to full-range overload reps with the cambered bench press bar and dumbbells.

A cambered bench press bar is a bar with a bend in it, which allows extra stretch while doing bench presses. It form-fits the chest when you lower it; the arms go down as far as possible with dumbbells, but the barbell allows you to use heavier weight. Combined with Dumbbell Bench Presses, you will improve your pressing strength through the greatest range of motion possible.

Cambered Bar Bench Press

Start with the Cambered Bar Bench Press, doing three to five sets of eight to four reps and increase weight as your reps go down. Pause the last rep of each set (let the bar sit on your chest, your body tight) for two seconds before blasting the final rep and mentally focusing on it as if you were attempting a max rep.

Keep the hand at the bend in the bar (shoulder width), increasing the stretch on the pecs even more.

Dumbbell Bench Press (decline bench)

Go next to palms-in Dumbbell Bench Presses on a decline bench, bringing the dumbbells back to the throat as far as possible and keeping the elbows back and out to the side. Do from six to 15 reps for five sets.

Flat Bench Flyes

Finish this stretch bench routine with Flat Bench Flyes, four to six sets of 8 to 12 reps for pectoral hypertrophy and a different type of stretch.

Cambered Bar Bench Press—3-5 sets 8-4 reps
Dumbbell Bench Press (palms in on decline bench)—5 sets of 15, 12, 10, 8, 6
Flat Bench Fly—4-6 sets 8-12 reps

Do this routine once a week or twice every 10 days.

POWER BENCH CYCLING FOR STRENGTH

Powerlifters, when training for an important contest, vary their reps according to how close they are to the date of competition. They know from years of research and practice that you cannot always be at the peak of your strength, and that to try to do so is to court injury.

Instead of trying to be at their

best all the time, they train in cycles, increasing the intensity and decreasing the volume of work done to maximize recovery. They also know that changing the rep scheme about once every three weeks shocks the body and produces new adaptations, the real purpose of training.

The body also reacts better if the change in reps is fairly large. Jumping from 10 reps a set to sets of explosive fives shocks the system more than dropping to eight reps, then sixes, then fours.

The exercises also change during the cycle, going from mostly isolation and bodybuilding training to a true powerlifting style. Assistance exercises are used more in the beginning of the cycle and less at the end.

The first three weeks use the Dumbbell Bench Press on the flat bench (palms in), the Incline (40 degree) Dumbbell Press (palms in) and Seated Dumbbell Shoulder Press (75 degree) for four to six sets of 10 reps each. Use a moderate cadence and minimal explosiveness. You're training for basic muscle size and joint strength in your adaptation, as well as deep ranges of motion. Finish the routine with Pressdowns and Hammer Curls, each for three sets of 10.

The second three weeks, switch to the Barbell Bench Press with a shoulder-width grip. Work for five sets of five, pausing the last rep of each set for two seconds. Use a power style on the bench, upper back arched, shoulder blades pulled tight.

The second exercise is the Dumbbell Incline Press on a 20-degree incline with palms facing away the entire set. This involves the shoulders more, readying them for the stress of heavy benches. Do five heavy sets of five here too, but with no pauses.

The third exercise is the Power Push-up on the floor. Pausing at the bottom of the push-up, blast off the floor as high as possible. Reposition yourself and go again. Do three sets of 10 reps.

The last three weeks of the cycle do Power Bench Presses (regular grip, if different); three sets of three with 90 percent of your max weight and five to 10 minutes rest between sets. Make sure you keep your shoulders warm. Give all the power and strength you can muster. Focus on bringing the bar down under control and then driving it off your chest with the upper torso.

After you finish these, go to Parallel Bar Dips and do four to six sets of as many Explosive Rep Dips as you can, using the same controlled negative, explosive-positive technique.

At the end of three weeks go for a single rep if you desire, but in this manner:

1×6 reps 80 percent max
1×3 reps 85 percent max
1×1 reps 90 percent max
1×1 reps 95 percent max
1×1 reps 105 percent max

This procedure will ensure that you are warmed up enough for the heavy weights, but not tired out. Work for the most perfect technique possible, especially on the lighter weights. Start the next cycle with 5 percent more weight on all exercises.

FIRST THREE WEEKS

	Sets	Reps
Flat Bench Dumbbell Bench Press (palms in)	4-6	10
40-degree Dumbbell Incline Press (palms in)	4-6	10
75-degree Seated Dumbbell Press (palms in)	4-6	10

SECOND THREE WEEKS

	Sets	Reps
Shoulder-Grip Barbell Bench Press	5	5
20-degree Dumbbell Incline Press (palms facing away)	5	5
Power Push-up	3	10

THIRD THREE WEEKS

	Sets	Reps
Power Bench Press (regular grip)	3	3
	(90 percent max)	
Explosive Dip	4-6	max

LAST DAY OF THREE WEEKS: NEW MAX

1×6 at 80 percent
1×3 at 85 percent
1×1 at 90 percent
1×1 at 95 percent
1×1 at 100 percent

STRENGTH/POWER ALTERNATE WORKOUT

Here is a combination routine for those who want to train their chest twice a week. The first workout is a basic strength workout focusing on the power bench and exercises for training the joint stabilizers. The second workout of the week is lighter and faster to develop the power and explosiveness necessary for big benches.

Start the first workout of the week with Flat Bench Barbell Benches. Do six sets of four and pause the last rep on each set for two seconds. Raise the weight five pounds when you can do all six sets of four.

The next exercise is Flat Bench Fly, a movement that big Bill Kazmaier, who has benched 661 pounds, says was essential in giving him the pectoral size, strength and development to increase his bench from 300 to 500 pounds. He says that after he did 5×5 with 525 pounds, and 4×5 with 550 pounds, then 452 pounds with a wide then narrow grip for three sets of 10, assistance exercises for the pecs were no longer necessary.

Do four to six sets of six to eight reps in the flyes.

Next turn to the Lying Triceps Press with the EZ curl bar. Instead of lowering the bar to the forehead as is traditionally done, let the elbows move forward toward the hips as the bar descends to your upper chest. The movement is basically the same as the Lying Triceps Extension, except that more weight can be used and it doesn't hurt your elbows.

On the next chest workout day (three to four days later) focus on "explosiveness training" for the chest, using fairly light weights. The first exercise is speed reps on the Cam II Vertical Bench Press. Because very little stretch can be used in this exercise, we will focus on holding body position tight while driving the arms out as fast as possible. Do not resist the negative part of the rep. Focus on working the positive rep only.

Do as many reps as possible for 20 seconds. Have a training partner keep track of the time. Do four sets of Cam II Vertical Bench Presses, keeping the weights up only if the speed does not diminish. Speed is the priority.

Power Chair Push-ups will work the range of motion that the vertical benches couldn't. Set up three chairs and do as many reps as possible in four 20-second periods. Do not let your body relax. This is a key component of speed training. You want to be able to work fast, but without losing form. If you have good explosive power but every time you drive the bar off your chest you break form, the explosiveness is not helping you.

Do Power Floor Dips to finish the speed and explosiveness session. Do the same rep and time scheme as the other exercises. In this section, keep the hands at shoulder width and the back flat. Touch your chest to the floor momentarily and then power off. Get in as many reps as you can in 20 seconds. Rest enough to fully recover between sets (this goes for all the exercises); one to one-and-a-half minutes should be adequate, because the training load will be light.

Cam II Vertical Bench Press 4 sets, 20 seconds of max reps

Power Chair Push-up 4 sets, 20 seconds of max reps

Power Floor Dip 4 sets, 20 seconds of max reps

MULTI-GROOVE BENCH PRESSING

One of the challenges of heavy bench pressing is keeping the bar in that elusive groove. The heavier the weights, the easier it is for the bar to slide up or down the chest, stressing the pecs and shoulders and usually causing a missed lift.

Training the bench press high on the chest, low on the chest and with a wide and narrow grip prepares the body and mind for any change in the bench press range of motion. It will be much easier to "pull one back" into the correct groove if your strength from multi-groove bench pressing is intact. This workout makes a perfect second-day training session for the chest, after doing regular heavy benches on the first day.

Start the workout with three sets of five in the Medium-Grip Bench Press to the neck. This provides maximum stretch while working the upper pectorals. Keep the elbows back in line with the shoulders as you press the weight up to help isolate the pecs.

Next do wide-grip benches to the lower pecs, working for sternal isolation. Again, do three sets of five, as heavy as possible. The elbows should be in line with the hands as you lower the bar.

The third exercise is narrow-grip benches to the mid-chest, working for triceps inner pec and shoulder isolation. Three sets of five will be enough.

The last exercise is wide-grip benches to the neck to work the entire pec region, especially the upper pecs and shoulders. Do three sets of five.

	Sets	Reps
Shoulder-Width Grip Bench Press to Neck	3	5
Wide-Grip Bench to Low Pecs	3	5
Narrow-Grip Bench Press	3	5
Wide-Grip Bench to Neck	3	5

With these exercises and principles to get you started, you should make strength gains from the first workout. Remember that you must train heavy to overload the muscles, and you must rest to grow. If you train hard enough, you will want to rest.

Strength training has so many practical applications in real life that it is perhaps the best weight training most people can do. Many people want to be able to do something with the muscles they get from hard bodybuilding training. Training the chest for strength and power provides that from the start.

TWELVE: SPEED TRAINING

Speed training is essential for all athletes. It not only conditions the body through the training required to establish and increase speed, but also increases joint strength, coordination and flexibility, and readies the body for athletic events. Sports themselves don't injure the body as much as the shock of subjecting a body to dynamic motion when it's not prepared.

For most athletic events, training for speed, power and coordination are vital to success. If a martial artist is very strong but cannot recruit the muscle fibers quickly enough to throw a lightning-fast punch, he has a weakness that makes him vulnerable.

A gymnast that is vaulting over the long horse must also have a chest that is properly speed-trained to make the most of his musculature. Natural speed is partly the result of genetic heritage, but it can be improved through training.

Train progressively in order to stimulate adaptation. Stress must be enough to overload the system and be as specific as possible. The easiest way to overload the speed mechanisms of the muscles is to do more work in the same or less amount of time. Keep the amount of time constant and try to increase the number of reps you do. You will need a watch with a second hand and a training partner to time you for best results in speed training.

The poundage will have to be light to work fast. Fifty percent of a 10-rep max is about right. If the load is too heavy, speed cannot be achieved.

Many sports require pushing motion from the upper body. As I've mentioned, gymnastics uses fast, explosive pushes in vaulting, parallel bar, rings, floor exercise and pommel horse. The only event that does not require fast upper-body movements is the horizontal or "high" bar.

Field athletes such as shot putters, javelin throwers, discus throwers and hammer throwers would benefit greatly from speed training their chest. For many throwers, lifting is a vital part of their training regimen. They train for explosion rather than just speed and utilize international (Olympic lifts) as well as the traditional bench presses in their weight work.

Although you should use mostly free weights in speed training, machine work allows you to concentrate on recruiting more muscles faster. It also helps reduce the risk of injury, as speed training is perhaps the easiest way to injure the joints; speedwork requires perfect form.

Machines allow you to discount the negative portion of the rep, something you cannot do with free weights. You have the opportunity to concentrate on the positive portion of the rep where speed is learned.

Cam II machines, which use air pressure for resistance, are perhaps the best for speed training, outside of isokinetic bench press machines, which are hard to find. Isokinetic machines allow you to set a precise rate of movement for the bar; the harder you push the more resistance is increased, but the bar continues to travel at the same speed.

When training for speed, you must have an extremely precise path of motion. Every inch you deviate from the most biomechanically correct movement slows your rate of travel. Visualizing the exact path you wish the bar to travel will improve performance. Imagery training as its called is used extensively by Russian athletes for increased efficiency and the mind/body connection.

More stress should not be applied to an area until it has fully recovered. If the area is trained before full recovery, it will not adapt as quickly and you could lose the adaptations you have previously stimulated, which is called overtraining.

The key to training is to listen to your body and adjust constantly to its changing capacities. In powerlifting, this is called free cycling, or to put it simply, going for it when you feel great. When you don't feel great you go for a little less. If you continue feeling poorly for a long time, you are probably overtrained. Take a week off and start again on a less severe program.

SPEED TRAINING ROUTINES

Cam II Pre-Exhaust Speed Training

This is an excellent way to reach deep into the fibers of the pecs for the most speed adaptations possible. Pre-exhausting the pecs with Cam II equipment involves going from the chest isolation machine (or pec dec) immediately to the vertical bench press.

Set the pressure gauge on a setting you know you can do 20 reps with. Using perfect form, do as many reps as possible for a set period of time. The time depends on where you are in your training. If you are just beginning speed training, go for 45-second intervals with 30-second rests. Do as many as possible on the chest machine before moving to the press.

As you become more fit, decrease the work interval to 30 seconds or even 20 seconds and take a full recovery after both exercises are completed. On the chest machine, focus on chest isolation, keeping the back flat against the bench and the hips on the seat. Focus on performing a fast positive rep and let the negative come back unresisted. Keep the entire body tight.

After three to five super-sets go to Floor Dips (push-ups) and do as many as possible for three bouts of 30 seconds. Tap the chest on the floor and for the best results, don't completely lock out the arms. Get into a rhythmic pumping action. Again, total body tightness is crucial.

Cam II Chest Machine and Cam II Vertical Bench Press 3-5 bouts of 30- to 45-second work intervals

Floor Dips 3 bouts of 30 seconds maximum reps

Multiangle Speed Push-up Routine

Here's a very easy workout you can do anywhere. By varying the elbow and body position during a push-up, you can adapt the entire chest and shoulder area to speedwork without weights.

Start the workout by performing Floor Dips with the elbows out, touching the solar plexus to the floor each rep; keep your head up and work for total pec isolation. Determine work and rest intervals by your present needs. If conditioning is a priority, or technique or strength, work for longer rest intervals and less lifting.

Keep the elbows in line with the shoulders as you do chest pushups. Strive for three to five sets.

Go next to Floor Dips with your feet on a chair or stool behind you and your elbows at a 45-degree angle from the body. Focus on using the upper chest and triceps to do most of the work. Three bouts lasting 30 to 60 seconds with 30 to 60 seconds rest will stimulate the chest muscles for speed.

Finish the routine with floor dips with the elbows tight against the body to isolate the shoulders and triceps. Keep the body rigid, the head in a neutral position. Contract the triceps strongly with each rep. Three bouts of 30 to 60 seconds should be enough for the pushing muscles of the torso.

Floor Dip (elbows out) 3 bouts of 30-60 seconds

Push-up

(feet up, elbows at 45 degrees) 3 bouts of 30-60 seconds

Close-Hand Triceps Push-up 3 bouts of 30-60 seconds

Power Pushing: Speed Training the Olympic Way

Weightlifters and power throwers usually train with the Olympic (now called international) lifts using heavy weights and an explosive style. The result is size, strength, speed and power. By using lighter weights you can obtain more reps, speed and a perfect explosive positive rep.

Because the upper torso is capable of producing power in so many ranges of motion, I have not limited this workout to just chest exercises, but also those shoulder pressing movements that involve the chest as well as shoulders.

You must be extremely cautious with this type of training to avoid injury; never drop the negative part of the rep or be sloppy about form. Use weight that you can do 15 strict but slow reps with and do the positive rep as explosively as possible, controlling and resisting the negative rep. With the standing push press, remember to never arch your back, but take up the stress with the quadriceps.

Standing Push Press

Start the routine with Standing Dumbbell Push Presses, dumbbells at shoulder level. Begin the overhead press by bending the knees slightly and coordinate pushing with the legs and arms. Finish the press at the three-quarter lockout position, your back strong and straight. Lower to the shoulders and repeat for maximum reps; do three sets.

Power Jerk

Next is the Power Jerk from the rack. Start the exercise with the barbell supported on a squat rack at shoulder level. Take the bar from the rack and stand straight with your legs slightly bent. With a strong thrust from the legs, drive the bar overhead to a lockout position and split the legs into a lunge. This is the finish position of the jerk

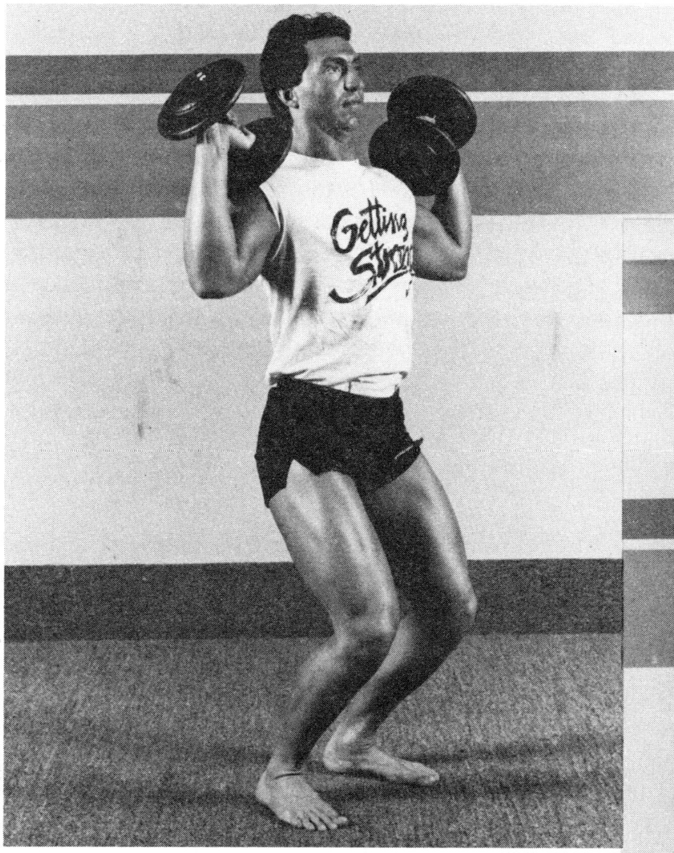

The Dumbbell Push Press begins with your knees bent and your elbows out to your sides. From here you push the dumbbells overhead using the power of your legs, shoulders and triceps.

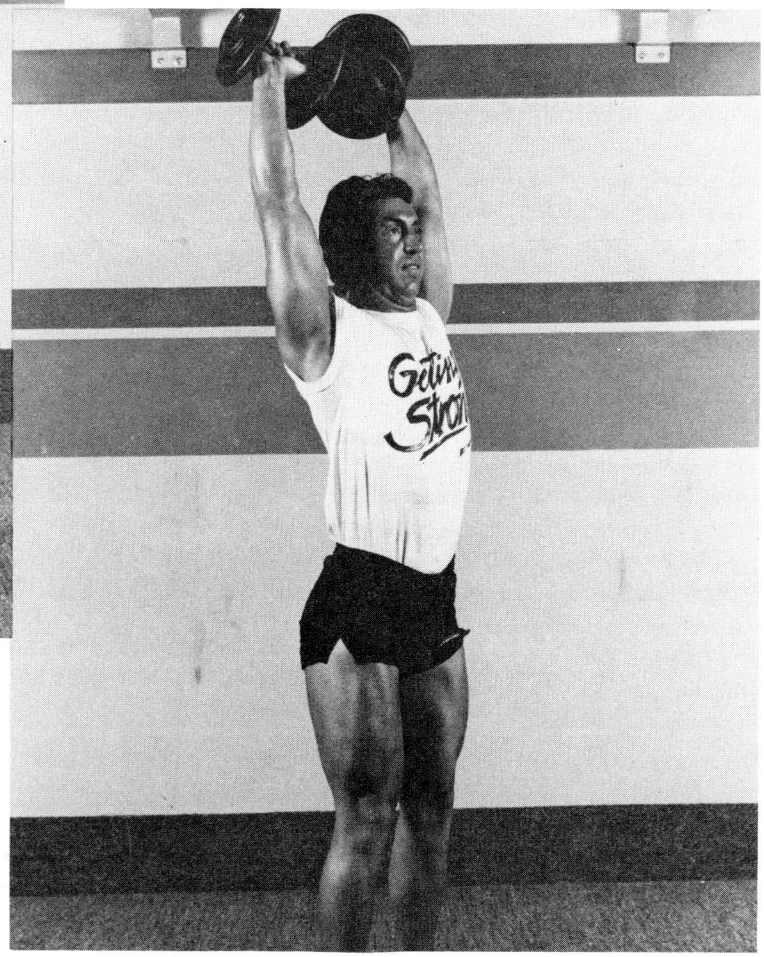

At the completion of the Dumbbell Push Press, the dumbbells should lightly touch each other.

portion of the clean and jerk and requires tremendous speed, coordination and balance. Such training is well suited for athletes whose sport requires speed and strength, like football, gymnastics or shot putting. Do three sets of 15 reps.

Flat Bench Explosive Press

Finish the workout with power Bench Presses on a flat bench using the same technique: slow negative reps followed by explosive positive reps. Do three sets of 15.

Make sure you hang from a chinning bar and stretch the lower back out, because this workout stretches the spinal cord.

	Sets	Reps
Standing Push Press	3	15
Power Jerk (from rack)	3	15
Flat Bench Explosive Press	3	15

This routine would also be very effective if you did all the reps as fast as possible, but varied the rep scheme for each exercise. You might do three sets of eight for the first, 3 sets of 10 for the second and 3 sets of 15 for the third. You can also vary the rep for each exercise, rotating each workout.

Speed Dipping

This is one of the hardest and most effective chest routines for speed. Speed Dipping is similar to the multiangle floor dip routine, but parallel bar dips are used instead of push-ups. The results are much more dramatic because the exercise is much more difficult to perform.

You must master the basic dipping position for chest isolation, the power dip (a combination exercise) and triceps isolation dips. Training for speed requires that the movement be as automatic and as technically perfect as possible.

Start the routine with chest isolation dips. Put your elbows out to your sides, back rounded, chin on the chest (even on the positive reps) and feet forward of the body as you dip. Control the negative rep, going for a full, deep stretch and then explode through the pecs, rising as fast as possible. Thinking about speed as you start the positive rep helps more than you might think. Stay with this exercise for three sets of as many reps as possible.

Take a three-minute rest after three sets. Go to Triceps Isolation Dips, keeping the head up, the chest high and feet behind the body. Do three sets of max reps. You should be tired by now, so make each rep count.

After a 5- to 10-minute rest go to power dips using both chest and triceps to complete the movement. Lower with the pecs, leaning into the movement and keeping the chest isolation positions, but with the elbows pinned to your sides for best leverage. Keep the back round and chin down as you contract your triceps as fast as possible for the positive rep. Three sets of max reps should take care of your chest training for the day.

VARIED ANGLE, RHYTHMIC PUMPING SPEED TRAINING

Bodybuilders who use pumping as their main training technique learn to move great amounts of weight for many repetitions with this style of training. It won't get you absolute speed but it will condition the chest to train faster with fewer wasted motions on traditional bodybuilding exercises.

The routine also takes the pecs through a full range of motion with this speed training, starting at horizontal with flat bench presses, going to 45-degree presses, and bringing more shoulder into the workout with 75-degree incline presses. The program finishes with vertical push presses with a barbell. Combining speed training through all these ranges of motion gets deep into the pecs, shoulders and triceps.

Use weights that allow 15 good reps and focus on keeping the dumbbell or barbell moving at all times. Go for a non-lock finish position and a smooth pistonlike action, three to five sets.

Flat Bench Press With Barbell

Begin with flat bench presses with a barbell. This allows you to concentrate more on a fast positive rep and less on balance than would dumbbells. Tap the chest lightly (don't bounce) and finish at three-quarters lockout.

Palms Away Dumbbell Incline Press

Go next to Palms Away Dumbbell Incline Presses on a 45-degree incline. Press the dumbbells smoothly up and down and try to get the 15 reps done as smooth as possible.

On the 75-degree dumbbell incline presses, keep the palms facing away to derive the most strength and muscle involvement possible. This is essentially a shoulder press but the upper pecs are heavily involved.

Standing Dumbbell Push Press

Finish the workout with Standing Dumbbell Push Presses with a bit of help from the legs; coordinate with the shoulder pushing motion. You are trying to get the whole body to work as a unit with this one.

	Sets	Reps
Flat Bench Barbell Press	3-5	15
Dumbbell Incline Press (45-degree bench)	3-5	15
Dumbbell Incline Press (75-degree bench)	3-5	15
Standing Dumbbell Push Press	3-5	15

Numerous activities and movements can train the chest for improved speed very effectively. These can used in addition to or as the main thrust of the weight workout. They add variety to the workout and allow you to use the muscles you've built up so much.

Medicine Ball Throwing

Don't laugh. Throwing a medicine ball is very hard. Two people can speed train the chest quickly and efficiently by sitting with their feet straight in front of them and throwing the ball to one another. When you catch the ball, roll backward as if you were going to do a back roll, letting your feet roll off the ground until they are vertical. Roll back now and simultaneously push the medicine ball to your partner as fast and explosively as possible. Do this as long as you can.

Rubber Pulleys or the Inner Tube Method to a Fast Chest

Cut a bicycle inner tube in half. As you stretch it, you're almost developing an isokinetic motion because no negative resistance is encountered. Gymnasts do this workout to develop reflexes.

Attach the middle of the inner tube securely to a wall behind you with both ends in your hands. Walk forward until the arms are almost behind you and the slack is out of the inner tube. Do these like very fast Cable Crossovers, bringing the hands out in front of you as fast as possible through a semicircular motion. Return to the start position immediately and do as many reps as possible for various lengths of time. For short bursts of speed use shorter work intervals. For endurance do longer work intervals.

Wall Pushoff

This is another gymnastic drill used to isolate and speed train the pushing muscles for tumbling and vaulting. The hardest part of this drill is trying not to fall over backward after each pushoff.

Start the exercise by leaning against a wall, your hands in a push-up position, fingers turned slightly in. Your body should be at approximately a 40- to 50-degree angle, depending on your arm

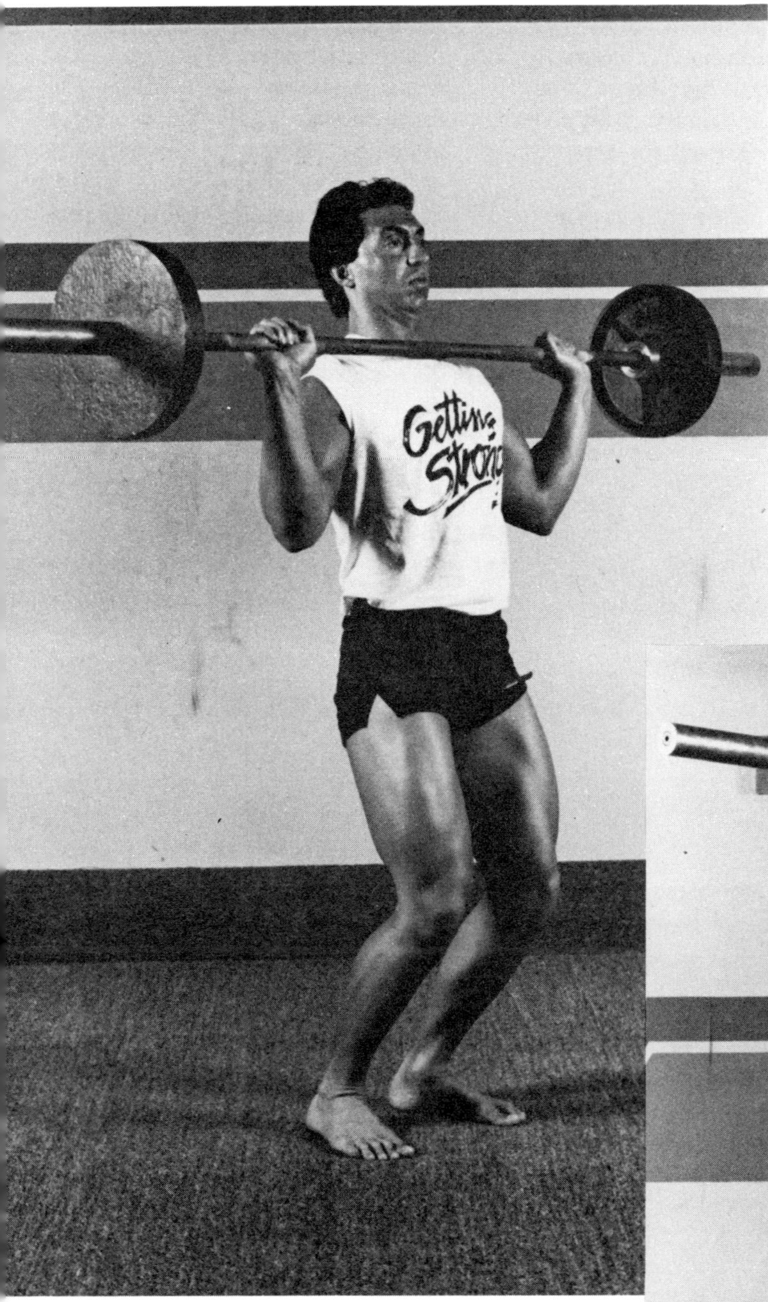

The Barbell Push Press begins with your knees bent and your elbows down. From here you push the barbell overhead using the strength from your legs, shoulders and triceps.

At the completion of the Barbell Push Press your arms should be fully extended.

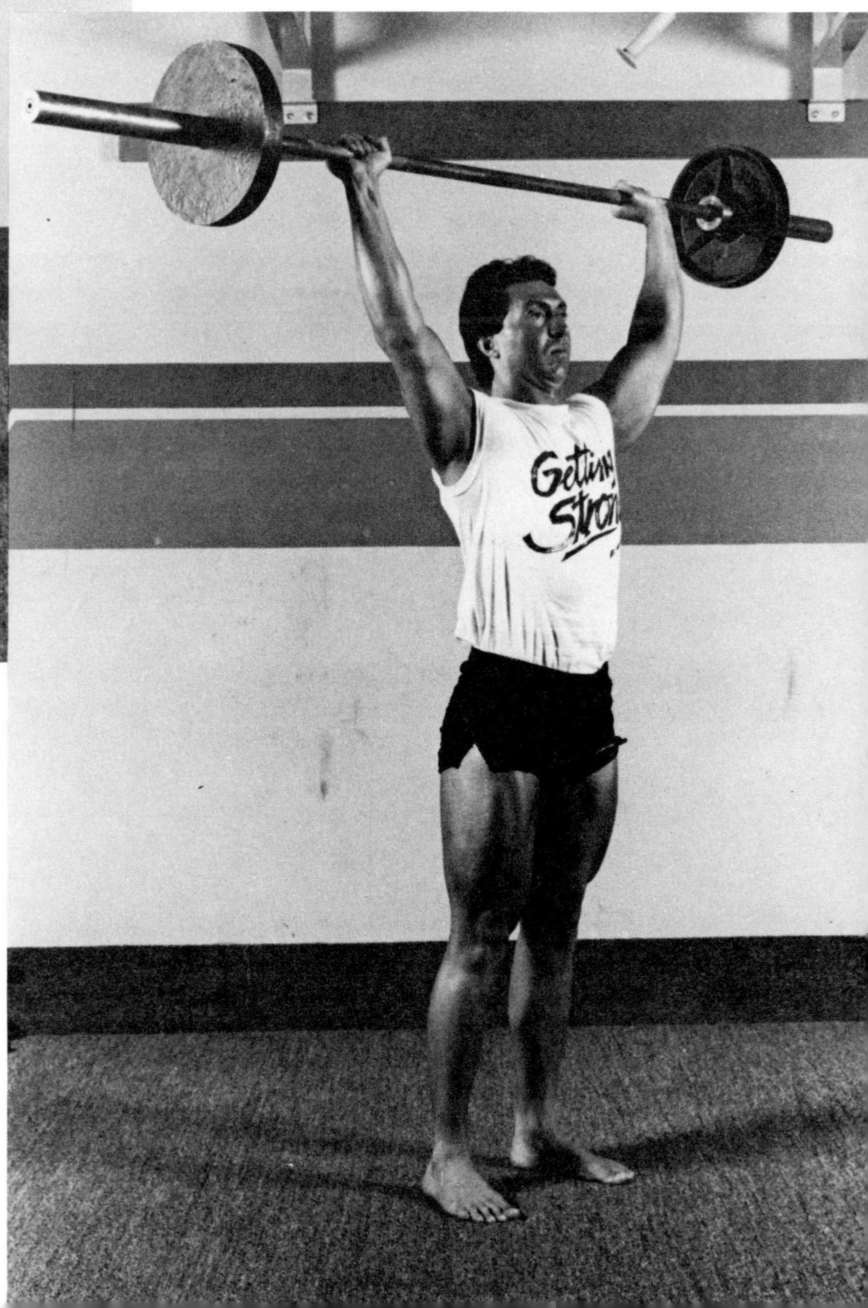

length. Lean into the wall slowly, positioning yourself. When you get as close as possible without touching, push off as fast as you can, then stop the push immediately. You are training for the initial reaction, the first section of the push. If you continue the push, you will undoubtedly land on your posterior.

When done correctly, the Wall Pushoff will bring your body back to a vertical position. Lean back into the wall and repeat for as many reps as you can. When the push becomes slow and uncoordinated, stop and rest. Repeat for three to five sets.

Speed training the chest is probably the most effective training method between heavy, high-intensity training cycles. Speed training goes well with strength training as it is such an important part of developing great strength. The more explosive you can be, the more muscle fibers you can reach and the stronger you can get. This is also a good time to give the body a rest from pushing heavy weights. After three to four weeks of speed training, your bench press will probably go up because you have improved your technique.

THIRTEEN: ENDURANCE TRAINING

Like strength or speed training, endurance training for the chest requires specific kinds of stress. The principle concept in endurance training is to progressively increase the duration of the activity rather than the resistance of the activity.

Running is perhaps the most familiar example of progressive endurance training. When you started running you probably could go for a mile or even less without stopping. You would run the same distance every day, though, working hard to go farther. After a week or more, you were running farther without stopping. If you continued training, you discovered that you continued to increase your running distance, as long as you ran a reasonable pace and didn't go into oxygen debt.

The time spent training was increased but the resistance remained the same, or even grew smaller, meaning you lost body fat (look on it as carrying weights). Although this certainly makes running easier, most of your improvement can be attributed to improved cardiovascular condition, not less weight.

The relationship between workload and duration is: the greater the workload (or resistance) the less time it can be maintained. The higher the intensity, the less duration. The two concepts are mutually exclusive. As Mike Mentzer, whose intense training style has set new standards for intensity training, says, you can sprint a hundred yards but you can't sprint a mile.

Because you always get what you train for, you must be very specific about how long you want your chest to perform and tailor your endurance program for the proper adaptation. Training your chest to endure an hour boxing match requires different training than for swimming the English Channel, although both require considerable pectoral and deltoid endurance. Generally, the longer the event the less intensity and the greater frequency and total training time required.

Remember, though, even when training for an endurance adaptation, base level strength is important. The greater your absolute strength level, the less low-intensity activity will deplete it.

MITOCHONDRIA: STOREHOUSES OF ENERGY

Mitochondria are the storehouses of energy in the cell. They process food into the product that your body makes energy from. They can take up to 30 percent of cell space and can increase in size and number when exposed to the stress of low-intensity, red-fiber training. The red fibers, or slow-twitch fibers, are the main storage areas for the mitochondria. This is the drumstick of the chicken, which is the dark meat. The chicken uses its legs constantly during the day for walking. The white fast-twitch fibers of the chicken's breast are rarely used for high-intensity work, like flapping the wings.

The muscle density and hardness that results from endurance training is partly the result of an increase in mitochondria size and number in the cells. The more demand you create for them, through aerobic low-intensity training, the greater their proliferation. This is one way the body builds endurance, by gradually increasing the mitochondria in the muscles.

With endurance training you also increase the proliferation of capillaries, the network of blood vessels that feed and supply the muscles with nutrients and blood to help promote growth and healing.

Regular endurance training can help prevent injuries, promote better circulation and local muscle endurance, as well as increase cardiovascular fitness. Interestingly, the arms burn calories more rapidly than the legs, making upper-body endurance exercise a priority for anyone concerned with losing body fat.

As noted in a previous chapter, the spot reducing theory has been denounced by almost everyone as bunk, but I haven't seen too many fat chests on gymnasts and wrestlers who constantly use their chests for long periods of time while training.

Swimming may be the endurance sport that uses the pecs most. Each stroke brings the chest muscles into play, especially the crawl. Remember, the main function of the pecs is to draw the arms down and across the body, as in the crawl. You can use swimming as a chest endurance workout, as well as build chest endurance by training the chest with weights.

Canoeing is another sport that requires chest endurance, as does its brethren kayaking. Look at a canoer's or kayaker's upper body. It's almost always very muscular and lean.

Gymnasts use their chests extensively in training but usually more in an anaerobic fashion similar to weight training, especially in competition. They do a great deal of endurance work in their daily workouts, though, where the chest and shoulders get used almost continuously. Gymnasts probably have the most defined and muscular pecs of any athletes, besides competitive bodybuilders.

Boxers use their chests for long periods of time, to hold their arms up in the fighting stance as well as to throw punches. Crossing the arms in front of the chest brings the pecs into the motion.

Light Loads, Long Duration

The greater the intensity of a movement, the more effort required, and the less time it can be performed. Short bursts of effort require a high-octane fuel, so to speak, which the body provides during anaerobic (without oxygen) work in the form of glycogen (sugar).

The endurance athlete wishes to keep going for long periods of time, so the load must be lighter so that more repetitions can be performed. Intensity levels must be moderate (50 percent of max or less) and the work performed continuously for long periods of time. This is aerobic (with oxygen) work and is the basis for endurance training.

The type of fuel used is dependent on the intensity of the activity. The body can choose between sugar and fat and a combination of both for most types of work. The lighter the load and the longer the work performed, the more fat is used for fuel. After two hours of low-intensity work, up to 90 percent of the fuel is stored fat reserves. The shorter and more explosive the activity, the more sugar is used for fuel. If you want your chest to perform for long periods of time, you must adapt it to using fat as an energy source by doing increasing amounts of work at the same level of intensity. Once you have reached the duration you want to perform at, then you increase the resistance while keeping the duration constant.

Rest Periods

Endurance work is defined as continuous work done for a prolonged period of time. For your chest to adapt, you must work it with less and less rest between sets until it is capable of performing for long periods of time with little or no rest. You can monitor your pulse to be sure you maintain an aerobic workout (75 percent of maximum heart rate) or you can use the much simpler but effective talk test. If you can carry on a conversation while you are performing, you are working aerobically. I have found that I do not have to talk to find this level. Just being able to think clearly while I am exercising usually always leaves me in the "target zone" for increasing endurance.

EXERCISE SELECTIONS

The chest muscles are hardly ever used to the exclusion of all other muscles; you also use the deltoids and triceps. Your training should reflect this and be as specific as possible, utilizing many compound movements as the foundation of your endurance training. You should teach the upper body to function with endurance in mind, shifting the load from muscle to muscle as the area gets fatigued.

Isolation exercises, however, will raise the pecs' absolute level of endurance. When the pecs become fatigued from isolation endurance exercises, the pace will have to slowed or the resistance lightened, as other muscles cannot pitch in and keep the pecs going. Both compound and isolation exercises are necessary for complete pectoral endurance adaptation.

Equipment Selection

Because the pectorals constitute such a small area of muscle, the more exercises you use for endurance training, and the more diverse the angle from which you train them, the greater the chest's adaptation. Use free weights, no weights, dipping bars, cables, machines, and any other available training devices. You do not have to concern yourself with spotters or having enough weights, so endurance training can be done almost anywhere at any time.

Training Frequency

The less intense an exercise, the more frequently you can do it. When training for chest endurance, you need to work the muscle more often. Runners train daily and sometimes twice a day. Because the area we are working is small, daily workouts aren't necessary, but three workouts a week is not excessive for endurance training.

Very low-intensity chest training such as swimming or walking with hand weights can be done daily up to for hours at a time. This type of high-rep endurance training, coupled with slightly higher intensity endurance weight training brings spectacular endurance adaptations!

Circuit Chest Training

The easiest way to endurance train the chest is with a circuit of different chest exercises that you do with little or no rest between sets. Train by time, working each station for 30 to 40 seconds; try for as may reps as possible, but keep the pace aerobic. Alternate the exercises to avoid burning out one section of muscle fibers too soon.

Universal Bench Press, Cable Cross, Parallel Bar Dip

Start the giant set with Bench Presses on a Universal machine. Use a wide grip to isolate the pecs as much as possible. The next exercise in the circuit is single-arm Cable Crosses, working one arm for 30 seconds, then the other. This lets the muscles assisting the chest rest a bit. Go to the third exercise, Parallel Bar Dips, and crank out as many as possible, using the power dip style.

Incline Press, Floor Dip

Incline presses on the shoulder pressing station of the Universal machine switches the stress to the upper pecs and delts, giving the lower pecs a little rest, but working the pecs hard. Drop to the floor after the incline and pump out as many floor dips as possible, using your knees for support when you become fatigued.

Straight-Arm Dumbbell Pullover

Finish the giant set with Straight-Arm Dumbbell Pullovers lying lengthwise on an exercise bench. This uses the lats to finish the pecs. Rest as little as possible and start the circuit over. Do as many circuits as necessary for your specific endurance time requirements.

The exercises I've just mentioned constitute one circuit. Do as many as necessary with enough rest between exercises to keep your pulse aerobic (75 percent of age-adjusted maximum heart rate).

PRE-EXHAUST GIANT SETS

Pre-exhaust technique involves alternating an isolation exercise with a compound exercise. The pecs do continuous work, but the smaller helping muscles of the triceps and shoulders have more recovery time.

Start the giant set with Flat Bench Dumbbell Flyes for 30 seconds; do as many reps as possible. Put down the dumbbells and go directly to Vertical Bench Presses on a Cam II machine. Doing the compound exercises on a machine will eliminate any balance problems and let you concentrate on contraction. Finish the 30 seconds and go back to Nautilus pec dec, again for 30 seconds. After the pec dec, use the pressing part of the Nautilus double chest to finish the pre-exhaust giant set. This is a very strenuous method of endurance training, so be careful and keep the loads light until you adapt.

Flat Bench Dumbbell Fly
Vertical Bench Press (Cam II)
Nautilus Pec Dec
Nautilus Decline Bench Press

This equals one giant set. Do as many as necessary according to the duration of the endurance goal.

GIANT SET MULTIJOINT EXERCISES

This workout is a killer! The shoulders and the triceps never get to rest the tension on the upper torso and the total workload is very high. At least the giant set travels from the top of the pecs to the bottom, isolating different sections as the exercises change. Use weights that you can handle with good form.

Parallel Bar Dip

Start with Parallel Bar Dips, using the power style to get the hardest exercise out of the way first. Don't worry about work intervals on this one; just do as many reps as possible.

Incline and Decline Press on Universal, Floor Dip

Go next to the Incline Press on the Universal machine, transferring the stress to the upper pecs and delts. Do 30 seconds of work. Go back down to the lower pecs with Decline Presses on the Universal machine for 30 seconds. Hit the mid-pecs with Floor Dips, elbows out and working for pec isolation. Forget time and do as may reps as possible.

Incline Press (45-degree)

Finish this giant set with Incline Presses at a 45-degree angle for 30 seconds. Rest as little as necessary and do three to five more giant sets.

Parallel Bar Power Dip (as many reps as possible)
Incline Press on Universal (30 seconds, max reps)
Decline Press on Universal Bench Press (30 seconds max reps)
Floor Dip (as many reps as possible)
45-degree Dumbbell Incline Press (30 seconds max reps)

ISOLATION GIANT SETS

For those masochists who relish hard work and a lot of it, isolation giant sets were made to order. Keeping the stress continuously on the pecs, there is literally no escape from the stress as the pecs get weaker and you go from exercise to exercise. As with the compound-exercise-only routine, the workload is shifted from upper to lower pecs to take some of the heat off. It doesn't help much!

Polaris Pec Dec, Bentover Cable Crossover

Start the workout with Polaris Pec Dec, hitting the entire pec area. Keep a rhythmic pumping action, not holding the peak contraction (you wouldn't get many reps if you did). Go for 60 seconds, really warming up the pecs. Next, go to the upper pecs with Bentover Cable Crossovers, crossing the hands in front of you at the finish. Do as many reps as you can in 45 seconds.

Upright Cable Crossover

Work the middle pecs with Upright Cable Crossovers. Stand up after the bentover cable work and continue the pumping. I told you this was going to be fun, right? Do 30 seconds of work on upright cable crossovers.

Polaris Crusher Pec Dec, Cross Bench Bent-Arm Dumbbell Pullover

Go directly to the Polaris Crusher Pec Dec to train the lower sections of the pecs. Twenty seconds of work should bring the blood down into the lower sections. Note that with each exercise the workload decreases so you can continue working with the same intensity throughout the giant set. Finish the giant set with Cross Bench Bent-Arm Dumbbell Pullovers, tilting the dumbbell forward on the positive reps to emphasize pec involvement.

Polaris Pec Dec, 60 seconds
Bent Cable Crossover, 45 seconds
Upright Cable Crossover, 30 seconds
Polaris Crusher Pec Dec, 20 seconds
Cross Bench Dumbbell
Pullover (tilting), 20 seconds

This equals one giant set. Do the maximum number possible.

DIP ENDURANCE

Dips not only train the pecs for endurance but affect the entire torso. If there were only one exercise I could do for my entire upper body, I'd do Dips. The exercise takes the muscles through the widest range of motion of any exercise and works the muscles in the length contraction and mid-range contraction position. By varying body and arm position, new exercises are created, isolating different sections of the chest and torso.

Varying the resistance, as when moving from Bar Dips to Floor Dips, keeps the dipping motion going for a long time. This routine takes it one step farther, changing the resistance slightly with each exercise, moving from hardest to easiest very gradually.

Each of the Dip exercises should be worked to momentary muscular failure to maximize the endurance effect. Take as little rest as possible between sets.

Parallel Bar Dip

Start the workout with the hardest dipping exercise, Parallel Bar Dips, using any style (chest isolation, triceps or power combination) for as many reps as possible.

Dips Between Chairs

Keep the range of motion full even when the bar dips give out by moving to Dips Between Chairs. Place your hands on two chairs and your feet on the third. Go for as long as you can. Finish the set with partial (top half) reps.

Floor Dip

The next exercise, Floor Dip, is even easier. Drop your knees on the ground and continue the pushing motion to take your pecs to new endurance levels. If you can't do Floor Dips, you can still keep the set going by using your knees to get you to the push-up position and just doing the negative reps for as long as possible.

TOTAL STRENGTH LEVEL ENDURANCE

Each person has at his command three different levels of strength to call on—positive, negative and static. Positive, or concentric strength, is the contraction responsible for shortening the muscle and raising weight. This is the weakest of the three strength levels.

After positive strength gives out, negative or eccentric strength takes over. Negative strength takes place when you lower weight and the muscle contracts while lengthening. This is the second strongest level of strength.

The strongest level of strength is static strength, where the muscle is locked into one position and holding weight.

One very effective method of increasing functional endurance is to take each of these three levels of strength to momentary muscular failure. Training for endurance requires increasing amounts of work, so always do as many sets and reps as you can.

Strength training on three levels is a very intense method of overloading the endurance part of the cell, which is why we will limit the routine to one exercise—Parallel Bar Dips. We do this because you can do the routine without assistance. The negatives are done by using a stool to raise yourself to the starting position and then resisting the negative rep.

If you have a good training partner, this routine can be done with his assistance to raise the weight after you reach positive failure. I like Dips, however, because the range of motion you get increases the difficulty and intensity.

Start the workout with power-style Dips using as much of the upper torso as possible. Go with a pumping style and try to get as much work done as quickly as possible. When you can't do any more, do half-reps only, pushing from the bottom as high up as possible.

When no more can be done, jump off the bars and take five very deep breaths. Next, use the stool to get to the top position and do negative reps for as long as possible. Each rep should take approximately two seconds to lower. Do not drop these; you can injure your shoulder quite easily if you do.

When you hit negative-rep failure, take 10 deep breaths and jump to the top position of the exercise; lower halfway down and hold for three seconds. Do this until you cannot even lock out your arms.

Beginners should not do this workout, because it is too intense. Intermediate-level trainers can do two sets and advanced trainers three. This one will make you very sore, so I advise everyone to start very easily and build up. After three or four weeks doing this workout, you will be amazed at how many more reps and sets you can do.

Since this is a high-intensity training technique, do this routine only two times per week.

Power Dips to Positive Failure
Power Dips to Negative Failure
Power Dips to Static Failure

This equals one set. Begin with one and work up slowly.

SIX-DAY SUPER ENDURANCE ROUTINE

If you are training for a very long endurance event that utilizes the chest in a direct manner, such as ultra-distance swimming, you will benefit immensely from endurance training the chest daily.

The easiest method of doing this routine is to start by using the total strength endurance routines three days per week. Alternate routines each workout. Do this for two weeks. For the next two weeks, continue alternating different endurance workouts, but add one more for a total of four chest endurance workouts in one week. Do two days on, a day off, two days on, two days off.

In the next two weeks, go to a five-day split, working the chest five days straight before taking a two-day rest. Some very low-intensity work such as slow swimming would be good exercise for the two rest days. Keep switching the routines daily, never giving the chest a chance to fully adapt to the varying endurance workloads.

After the final two weeks of five days, go to a six-day routine, doing all of the workouts once a week. Change the starting order each week. Do this for the next four weeks, by which time you should be capable of keeping your pecs contracting forever!

Endurance training is an integral part of a complete and balanced bodybuilding program, and it has many benefits: cardiovascular equal to running or any aerobic program, a lower percentage of body fat, lower resting pulse rate, stronger more efficient heart, greater resistance to pain, and less fatigue and illness.

A sense of pace and rhythm are fringe benefits of high-rep training, as well as an increased production of endorphins, chemicals produced in the brain that have been associated with the "exercise high."

Rotating the type of training, shaping routines, definition and endurance routines will train your chest with every possible angle and with every conceivable technique.

Rotating workouts will also help keep you mentally fresh and reduce injuries from doing too much of one type of training for too long. Training for strength is excellent, but too much will result in tendon and joint pain. The same can be said about every type of training.

BEGINNING CHEST ROUTINE

EXERCISE	RECOMMENDED SETS × REPS	SETS × REPS PERFORMED	MAXIMUM POUNDAGES MON	WED	FRI
WEEK 1					
Full Breathing Squat	1×20				
Barbell Straight Arm Pullover	1×20				
Barbell Bench Press	3×20				
Dumbbell Pullover	3×12				
WEEK 2					
Full Breathing Squat	2×20				
Barbell Straight Arm Pullover	2×20				
Barbell Bench Press	3×20				
Dumbbell Pullover	3×12				
WEEK 3					
Full Breathing Squat	2×20				
Barbell Straight Arm Pullover	2×20				
Barbell Bench Press	3×20				
Dumbbell Pullover	3×12				
WEEK 4					
Full Breathing Squat	2×20				
Barbell Straight Arm Pullover	2×20				
Barbell Bench Press	3×20				
Dumbbell Pullover	3×12				
WEEK 5					
Full Breathing Squat	3×20				
Barbell Straight Arm Pullover	3×20				
Barbell Bench Press	3×20				
Dumbbell Pullover	3×12				

ADVANCED BASIC ROUTINE

EXERCISE	RECOMMENDED SETS × REPS	SETS × REPS PERFORMED	MAXIMUM POUNDAGES MON	WED	FRI
WEEK 1					
45-Degree Incline Barbell Press	3×15,12,10				
Flat Bench Fly	3×15,12,10				
10-Degree Incline Dumbbell Press	3×15,12,10				
Nautilus Pec Dec	3×15,12,10				
WEEK 2					
45-Degree Incline Barbell Press	3×15,12,10				
Flat Bench Fly	3×15,12,10				
10-Degree Incline Dumbbell Press	3×15,12,10				
Nautilus Pec Dec	3×15,12,10				
WEEK 3					
45-Degree Incline Barbell Press	3×15,12,10,8				
Flat Bench Fly	3×15,12,10,8				
10-Degree Incline Dumbbell Press	3×15,12,10,8				
Nautilus Pec Dec	3×15,12,10,8				
WEEK 4					
45-Degree Incline Barbell Press	3×15,12,10,8				
Flat Bench Fly	3×15,12,10,8				
10-Degree Incline Dumbbell Press	3×15,12,10,8				
Nautilus Pec Dec	3×15,12,10,8				
WEEK 5					
45-Degree Incline Barbell Press	3×15,12,10,8,6				
Flat Bench Fly	3×15,12,10,8,6				
10-Degree Incline Dumbbell Press	3×15,12,10,8,6				
Nautilus Pec Dec	3×15,12,10,8,6				

INVERTED PYRAMID ROUTINE

EXERCISE	RECOMMENDED SETS × REPS	SETS × REPS PERFORMED	MAXIMUM POUNDAGES MON	WED	FRI
WEEK 1					
Flat Bench Barbell Press	3×15,12,10				
Weighted Fly	3×15,12,10				
Flat Bench Fly	3×15,12,10				
WEEK 2					
Flat Bench Barbell Press	3×15,12,10				
Weighted Fly	3×15,12,10				
Flat Bench Fly	3×15,12,10				
WEEK 3					
Flat Bench Barbell Press	3×15,12,10,8				
Weighted Fly	3×15,12,10,8				
Flat Bench Fly	3×15,12,10,8				
WEEK 4					
Flat Bench Barbell Press	3×15,12,10,8				
Weighted Fly	3×15,12,10,8				
Flat Bench Fly	3×15,12,10,8				
WEEK 5					
Flat Bench Barbell Press	3×15,12,10,8,6				
Weighted Fly	3×15,12,10,8,6				
Flat Bench Fly	3×15,12,10,8,6				
WEEK 6					
Flat Bench Barbell Press	3×15,12,10,8,6				
Weighted Fly	3×15,12,10,8,6				
Flat Bench Fly	3×15,12,10,8,6				

BARBELL INVERTED PYRAMID ROUTINE

EXERCISE	RECOMMENDED SETS × REPS	SETS × REPS PERFORMED	MAXIMUM POUNDAGES MON	WED	FRI
WEEK 1					
Barbell Bench Press	3×15,12,10				
Barbell Incline Press	3×15,12,10				
Barbell Decline Press	3×15,12,10				
WEEK 2					
Barbell Bench Press	3×15,12,10				
Barbell Incline Press	3×15,12,10				
Barbell Decline Press	3×15,12,10				
WEEK 3					
Barbell Bench Press	3×15,12,10,8				
Barbell Incline Press	3×15,12,10,8				
Barbell Decline Press	3×15,12,10,8				
WEEK 4					
Barbell Bench Press	3×15,12,10,8				
Barbell Incline Press	3×15,12,10,8				
Barbell Decline Press	3×15,12,10,8				
WEEK 5					
Barbell Bench Press	3×15,12,10,8				
Barbell Incline Press	3×15,12,10,8				
Barbell Decline Press	3×15,12,10,8				

POWER FIVES WORKOUT

EXERCISE	RECOMMENDED SETS × REPS	SETS × REPS PERFORMED	MAXIMUM POUNDAGES MON	WED	FRI
WEEK 1					
Medium-Grip Barbell Bench Press	3×5				
Incline Dumbbell Press (40 degrees)	3×5				
WEEK 2					
Medium-Grip Barbell Bench Press	4×5				
Incline Dumbbell Press (40 degrees)	4×5				
WEEK 3					
Medium-Grip Barbell Bench Press	4×5				
Incline Dumbbell Press (40 degrees)	4×5				
WEEK 4					
Medium-Grip Barbell Bench Press	5×5				
Incline Dumbbell Press (40 degrees)	5×5				
WEEK 5					
Medium-Grip Barbell Bench Press	5×5				
Incline Dumbbell Press (40 degrees)	5×5				

SUPER-SET POST-EXHAUST WORKOUT

EXERCISE	RECOMMENDED SETS × REPS	SETS × REPS PERFORMED	MAXIMUM POUNDAGES MON	WED	FRI
WEEK 1					
Dumbbell Bench Press	3×15,12,10				
Dumbbell Fly	2×12,15				
WEEK 2					
Dumbbell Bench Press	3×15,12,10				
Dumbbell Fly	2×12,15				
WEEK 3					
Dumbbell Bench Press	3×15,12,10,8				
Dumbbell Fly	2×12,15				
WEEK 4					
Dumbbell Bench Press	3×15,12,10,8				
Dumbbell Fly	2×12,15				
WEEK 5					
Dumbbell Bench Press	3×15,12,10,8,6				
Dumbbell Fly	2×12,15				

UPPER PEC PRE-EXHAUST WORKOUT

EXERCISE	RECOMMENDED SETS × REPS	SETS × REPS PERFORMED	MAXIMUM POUNDAGES MON	WED	FRI
WEEK 1					
Incline Dumbbell Fly	2×12				
Incline Dumbbell Press	2×12				
Bentover Cable Crossover	2×15				
WEEK 2					
Incline Dumbbell Fly	2×12				
Incline Dumbbell Press	2×12				
Bentover Cable Crossover	3×15				
WEEK 3					
Incline Dumbbell Fly	3×12				
Incline Dumbbell Press	3×12				
Bentover Cable Crossover	3×15				
WEEK 4					
Incline Dumbbell Fly	3×12				
Incline Dumbbell Press	3×12				
Bentover Cable Crossover	4×15				
WEEK 5					
Incline Dumbbell Fly	3×12				
Incline Dumbbell Press	3×12				
Bentover Cable Crossover	4×15				

LOWER PEC TRI-SET WORKOUT

EXERCISE	RECOMMENDED SETS × REPS	SETS × REPS PERFORMED	MAXIMUM POUNDAGES MON	WED	FRI
WEEK 1					
45-Degree Decline Fly	2×12				
Standing Cable Crossover	2×12				
Narrow-Grip Bar Dip	2×12				
WEEK 2					
45-Degree Decline Fly	2×12				
Standing Cable Crossover	2×12				
Narrow-Grip Bar Dip	2×12				
WEEK 3					
45-Degree Decline Fly	3×12				
Standing Cable Crossover	3×12				
Narrow-Grip Bar Dip	3×12				
WEEK 4					
45-Degree Decline Fly	4×12				
Standing Cable Crossover	4×12				
Narrow-Grip Bar Dip	4×15				
WEEK 5					
45-Degree Decline Fly	4×12				
Standing Cable Crossover	4×12				
Narrow-Grip Bar Dip	4×12				
WEEK 6					
45-Degree Decline Fly	5×12				
Standing Cable Crossover	5×12				
Narrow-Grip Bar Dip	5×15				

ISOLATED COMPOUND EXERCISE SHAPING WORKOUT

EXERCISE	RECOMMENDED SETS × REPS	SETS × REPS PERFORMED	MAXIMUM POUNDAGES MON	WED	FRI
WEEK 1					
Barbell Bench Press to Throat	3×10				
Wide Bar Dip	3×MAX				
Low Incline Dumbbell Press	3×8				
WEEK 2					
Barbell Bench Press to Throat	4×10				
Wide Bar Dip	3×MAX				
Low Incline Dumbbell Press	3×8				
WEEK 3					
Barbell Bench Press to Throat	5×10				
Wide Bar Dip	4×MAX				
Low Incline Dumbbell Press	3×8				
WEEK 4					
Barbell Bench Press to Throat	5×10				
Wide Bar Dip	4×MAX				
Low Incline Dumbbell Press	3×8				
WEEK 5					
Barbell Bench Press to Throat	5×10				
Wide Bar Dip	4×MAX				
Low Incline Dumbbell Press	4×8				

MULTIANGULAR ISOLATION GIANT-SET WORKOUT

EXERCISE	RECOMMENDED SETS × REPS	SETS × REPS PERFORMED	MAXIMUM POUNDAGES MON	WED	FRI
WEEK 1 (Do 1 cycle)					
Standing Cable Cross	10 reps				
Nautilus Pec Dec	10 reps				
Cross Bench Dumbbell Pullover	10 reps				
Decline Fly	10 reps				
WEEK 2 (Do 2 cycles)					
Standing Cable Cross	10 reps				
Nautilus Pec Dec	10 reps				
Cross Bench Dumbbell Pullover	10 reps				
Decline Fly	10 reps				
WEEK 3 (Do 3 cycles)					
Standing Cable Cross	10 reps				
Nautilus Pec Dec	10 reps				
Cross Bench Dumbbell Pullover	10 reps				
Decline Fly	10 reps				
WEEK 4 (Do 3 cycles)					
Standing Cable Cross	12 reps				
Nautilus Pec Dec	12 reps				
Cross Bench Dumbbell Pullover	12 reps				
Decline Fly	12 reps				
WEEK 5 (Do 3 cycles)					
Standing Cable Cross	15 reps				
Nautilus Pec Dec	15 reps				
Cross Bench Dumbbell Pullover	15 reps				
Decline Fly	15 reps				

ALTERNATING PRE-EXHAUST GIANT-SET WORKOUT

EXERCISE	RECOMMENDED SETS × REPS	SETS × REPS PERFORMED	MAXIMUM POUNDAGES MON	WED	FRI
WEEK 1 (Do 2 cycles)					
Incline Dumbbell Fly	10 reps				
Incline Dumbbell Press	10 reps				
Flat Bench Fly	10 reps				
Flat Bench Dumbbell Press	10 reps				
Decline Fly	10 reps				
Decline Dumbbell Press	10 reps				
WEEK 2 (Do 2 cycles)					
Incline Dumbbell Fly	10 reps				
Incline Dumbbell Press	10 reps				
Flat Bench Fly	10 reps				
Flat Bench Dumbbell Press	10 reps				
Decline Fly	10 reps				
Decline Dumbbell Press	10 reps				
WEEK 3 (Do 2 cycles)					
Incline Dumbbell Fly	10 reps				
Incline Dumbbell Press	10 reps				
Flat Bench Fly	10 reps				
Flat Bench Dumbbell Press	10 reps				
Decline Fly	10 reps				
Decline Dumbbell Press	10 reps				
WEEK 4 (Do 3 cycles)					
Incline Dumbbell Fly	10 reps				
Incline Dumbbell Press	10 reps				
Flat Bench Fly	10 reps				
Flat Bench Dumbbell Press	10 reps				
Decline Fly	10 reps				
Decline Dumbbell Press	10 reps				

STRENGTH TRAINING WORKOUT

EXERCISE	RECOMMENDED SETS × REPS	SETS × REPS PERFORMED	MAXIMUM POUNDAGES MON	WED	FRI
WEEK 1					
Barbell Bench Press	3×10,8,6				
Narrow-Grip Bench Press	3×5				
Dip	3×MAX				
Dumbbell Hammer Curl	3×8				
WEEK 2					
Barbell Bench Press	4×10,8,6,6				
Narrow-Grip Bench Press	3×5				
Dip	3×MAX				
Dumbbell Hammer Curl	3×8				
WEEK 3					
Barbell Bench Press	4×10,8,6,6				
Narrow-Grip Bench Press	4×5				
Dip	3×MAX				
Dumbbell Hammer Curl	3×8				
WEEK 4					
Barbell Bench Press	4×10,8,6,6				
Narrow-Grip Bench Press	4×5				
Dip	4×MAX				
Dumbbell Hammer Curl	3×8				
WEEK 5					
Barbell Bench Press	4×10,8,6,6				
Narrow-Grip Bench Press	4×5				
Dip	4×MAX				
Dumbbell Hammer Curl	4×8				

DUMBBELL POWER BENCH WORKOUT

EXERCISE	RECOMMENDED SETS × REPS	SETS × REPS PERFORMED	MAXIMUM POUNDAGES MON	WED	FRI
WEEK 1					
Dumbbell Flat Bench Press	3×15,12,10				
Incline Dumbbell Press	3×15,12,10				
Chair Push-up	3×10,12				
Pressdown	3×10				
Dumbbell Front Raise	3×10				
Standing Dumbbell Lateral	3×10				
WEEK 2					
Dumbbell Flat Bench Press	4×15,12,10,8				
Incline Dumbbell Press	3×15,12,10				
Chair Push-up	3×10,12				
Pressdown	3×10				
Dumbbell Front Raise	3×10				
Standing Dumbbell Lateral	3×10				
WEEK 3					
Dumbbell Flat Bench Press	5×15,12,10,8,6				
Incline Dumbbell Press	4×15,12,10,8				
Chair Push-up	3×10,12				
Pressdown	3×10				
Dumbbell Front Raise	3×10				
Standing Dumbbell Lateral	3×10				
WEEK 4					
Dumbbell Flat Bench Press	5×15,12,10,8,6				
Incline Dumbbell Press	5×15,12,10,8,6				
Chair Push-up	3×10,12				
Pressdown	3×10				
Dumbbell Front Raise	3×10				
Standing Dumbbell Lateral	3×10				

CIRCUIT CHEST TRAINING FOR ENDURANCE

EXERCISE	RECOMMENDED SETS × REPS	SETS × REPS PERFORMED	MAXIMUM POUNDAGES MON	WED	FRI
WEEK 1 (Do 1 cycle for 30 seconds each exercise)					
Wide-Grip Universal Bench Press					
Single-Arm Cable Crossover					
Parallel Bar Dip					
Universal Incline Press					
Floor Dip					
WEEK 2 (Do 1 cycle for 40 seconds each exercise)					
Wide-Grip Universal Bench Press					
Single-Arm Cable Crossover					
Parallel Bar Dip					
Universal Incline Press					
Floor Dip					
WEEK 3 (Do 2 cycles for 30 seconds each exercise)					
Wide-Grip Universal Bench Press					
Single-Arm Cable Crossover					
Parallel Bar Dip					
Universal Incline Press					
Floor Dip					

(CONTINUED)

EXERCISE	RECOMMENDED SETS × REPS	SETS × REPS PERFORMED	MAXIMUM POUNDAGES MON	WED	FRI
WEEK 4 (Do 2 cycles for 40 seconds each exercise) *Wide-Grip Universal Bench Press*					
Single-Arm Cable Crossover					
Parallel Bar Dip					
Universal Incline Press					
Floor Dip					
WEEK 5 (Do 3 cycles for 30 seconds each exercise) *Wide-Grip Universal Bench Press*					
Single-Arm Cable Crossover					
Parallel Bar Dip					
Universal Incline Press					
Floor Dip					
WEEK 6 (Do 3 cycles for 40 seconds each exercise) *Wide-Grip Universal Bench Press*					
Single-Arm Cable Crossover					
Parallel Bar Dip					
Universal Incline Press					
Floor Dip					

POWER PUSHING FOR SPEED

EXERCISE	RECOMMENDED SETS×REPS	SETS×REPS PERFORMED	MAXIMUM POUNDAGES MON	WED	FRI
WEEK 1					
Standing Dumbbell Push Press	3×15				
Power Jerk From Rack	3×15				
Flat Bench Explosive Press	3×15				
WEEK 2					
Standing Dumbbell Push Press	4×15				
Power Jerk From Rack	3×15				
Flat Bench Explosive Press	3×15				
WEEK 3					
Standing Dumbbell Push Press	4×15				
Power Jerk From Rack	4×15				
Flat Bench Explosive Press	3×15				
WEEK 4					
Standing Dumbbell Push Press	4×15				
Power Jerk From Rack	4×15				
Flat Bench Explosive Press	4×15				

ABOUT THE AUTHOR

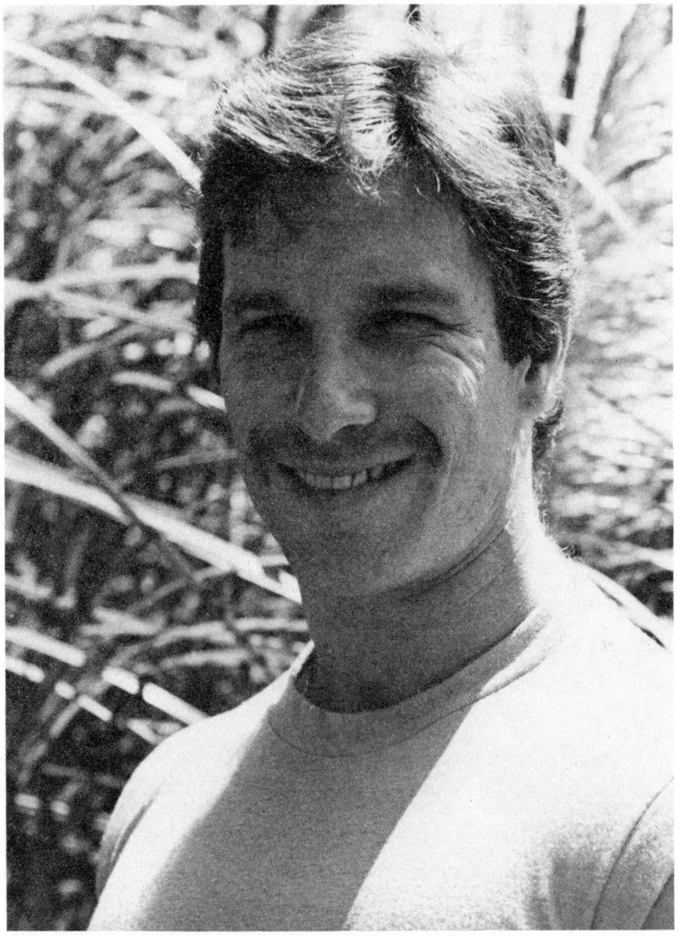

No one comes closer to fitting the description of renaissance athlete than Mark Reifkind. The author began his athletic career in gymnastics when he was 12 years old. While attending the University of Iowa, he was a nationally ranked gymnast. After college Reifkind broadened his athletic horizons, becoming an expert cyclist, racewalker and swimmer. For the past eight years the 27-year-old has concentrated on bodybuilding and working full-time as a private instructor. Reifkind lives in Palo Alto, California.